Pre-Hospital Obstetric Emergency Training

The Practical Approach

Advanced Life Support Group

EDITED BY

Malcolm Woollard

Kim Hinshaw

Helen Simpson

Sue Wieteska

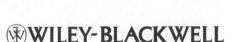

⊛WILEY-BLACKWELL

A John Wiley & Sons, Ltd., Publication

This edition first published 2010 © 2010 by Blackwell Publishing Ltd

BMJ Books is an imprint of BMJ Publishing Group Limited, used under licence by Blackwell Publishing which was acquired by John Wiley & Sons in February 2007. Blackwell's publishing programme has been merged with Wiley's global Scientific, Technical and Medical business to form Wiley-Blackwell.

Registered office: John Wiley & Sons Ltd, The Atrium, Southern Gate, Chichester, West Sussex, PO19 8SQ, UK

Editorial offices: 9600 Garsington Road, Oxford, OX4 2DQ, UK
  The Atrium, Southern Gate, Chichester, West Sussex, PO19 8SQ, UK
  111 River Street, Hoboken, NJ 07030-5774, USA

For details of our global editorial offices, for customer services and for information about how to apply for permission to reuse the copyright material in this book please see our website at www.wiley.com/wiley-blackwell

Library of Congress Cataloging-in-Publication Data

Pre-hospital obstetric emergency training : the practical approach / Advanced Life Support Group ; edited by Malcolm Woollard ... [et al.].
    p. ; cm.
  Includes bibliographical references and index.
  ISBN 978-1-4051-8475-5 (alk. paper)
  1. Obstetrical emergencies.   2. Emergency medical technicians.   I. Woollard, Malcolm.
II. Advanced Life Support Group (Manchester, England)
  [DNLM: 1. Obstetric Labor Complications–prevention & control.   2. Emergency Medical Services–methods.   3. Emergency Treatment–methods.   4. Health Personnel–education.
5. Inservice Training–methods. WQ 330 P9196 2009]
  RG571.P64 2009
  618.2′025–dc22

                                                                              2009009316

A catalogue record for this book is available from the British Library.

Set in 9/11.5pt Meridien by Aptara® Inc., New Delhi, India
Printed and bound in Singapore

1   2010

Contents

Note to text:
Drugs and their doses are mentioned in this text. Although every effort has been made to ensure accuracy, the writers, editors, publishers and printers cannot accept liability for errors or omissions. The final responsibility for delivery of the correct dose remains with the practitioner administering the drug.

Advanced
Life
Support
Group

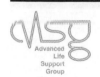

Advanced
Life
Support
Group

Contributors

Sally Evans	Midwifery, Middlesbrough
Kim Hinshaw	Obstetrics and Gynaecology, Sunderland
Helen Simpson	Obstetrics and Gynaecology, Middlesbrough
Mark Woolcock	Pre-Hospital Care, Truro
Malcolm Woollard	Pre-Hospital Care, Coventry
Jonathan Wyllie	Neonatology, Middlesbrough

Dedication

With thanks to our families for their tolerance and support during the development of this manual and its associated course.

Foreword

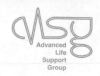

I was delighted and pleased to read 'POET' which gives practical advice to a range of practitioners. Although it is intended for pre-hospital practitioners there is valuable information for nurses, midwives, general practitioners (GPs) and pre- and post-registration doctors. The chapters cover a wide variety of topics starting from the organisation of obstetric services to details of anatomy, physiology and normal delivery. Once this is covered, the chapters logically proceed to a general approach to the obstetric patient followed by management of emergencies in early and late pregnancy and during delivery. The illustrations and flow charts of care pathways make it simple to read and to keep in mind the logical steps to be taken to provide the best care.

The chapter on 'Care of the baby at birth' is a welcome chapter for such a book. The management of non-obstetric emergencies, cardiac arrest and shock in pregnancy has different management issues compared with a woman who is not pregnant. The knowledge needed for these is provided in a way that could be easily understood. This chapter will be useful for a different range of practitioners.

POET is a comprehensive book that covers the knowledge needed for pre-hospital practitioners. But I would recommend this book for a wider audience of nurses, midwives, GPs and A&E doctors who may face the pregnant mother in an outside hospital setting or in a hospital with no maternity service provision. The authors deserve credit for simplifying a complex subject and for covering the knowledge needed on this topic for pre-hospital practitioners.

S. Arulkumaran FRCOG, PhD
Professor and Head of Obstetrics and Gynaecology
St George's University of London
November 2009

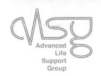

Preface

Pre-hospital obstetric incidents make up a significant proportion of the more costly litigation claims against UK ambulance services. These claims are based either on an alleged failure to identify and manage a problem or lack of appropriate equipment for the treatment of a preterm baby.

For a number of years after the UK national paramedic curriculum was introduced in the UK, it included no specific training on the management of obstetric emergencies at an 'advanced life support' level. Most staff received only a half-day of lectures during their initial ambulance technician training at the beginning of their career. Since 1999, advanced obstetrics and gynaecology became a mandatory part of the paramedic course for new entrants but with the expectation that existing paramedics would receive update training. Our experience has indicated, however, that paramedics in many parts of the UK have not had the opportunity to do so.

A confidential enquiry into maternal and child health (CEMACH) report has indicated that many of the pregnant women dying *'had chaotic lifestyles and found it hard to engage with maternity services'*. The ambulance service may be the initial contact with the health service for these patients and their peers who become unwell but are fortunate enough to survive. The CEMACH report identifies the need for a widened awareness of the risk factors and early signs and symptoms of potentially serious problems in pregnancy, and makes a number of key recommendations that could be addressed in part by appropriately trained pre-hospital practitioners. For example, it states:

All clinical staff must undertake regular, written, documented and audited training for:

- The identification, initial management and referral for serious medical and mental health conditions which, although unrelated to pregnancy, may affect pregnant women or recently delivered mothers
- The early recognition and management of severely ill pregnant women and impending maternal collapse

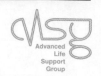

- The improvement of basic, immediate and advanced life support skills. A number of courses provide additional training for staff caring for pregnant women and newborn babies.

There is also a need for staff to recognise their limitations and to know when, how and whom to call for assistance.

This manual and its associated Advanced Life Support Group training course (also called POET) hope to meet these educational needs for a range of pre-hospital practitioners. Both the text and the course have been developed by a multi-disciplinary team of senior paramedics, consultant obstetricians and midwives, all of whom are practicing clinicians and experienced educators. POET course teaching teams have a similar multi-professional membership with a shared philosophy of combining pre-hospital and obstetric expertise. Although we anticipate that paramedics and pre-hospital physicians will make up the bulk of our readership and course candidates, POET will also be of value to nurses working in walk-in and unscheduled care centres and to midwives and to GPs – particularly those working at a distance from further support.

It is our sincere hope that POET will build the confidence and competence of pre-hospital practitioners and thus contribute to reducing the incidence of maternal and fetal mortality and morbidity.

Malcolm Woollard,
Helen Simpson,
Kim Hinshaw
and Sue Wieteska
November 2009

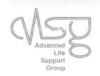
Advanced
Life
Support
Group

Acknowledgements

A great many people have worked hard to produce this book and the accompanying course. The editors thank all the contributors for their efforts and all POET providers and instructors who took the time to send their comments during the development of the text and the course, in particular Bernadette Norman who completed a full review of the text.

We also acknowledge Rachel Adams at ALSG for her support. We are also greatly indebted to Kate Wieteska for producing the first draft of the line drawings that illustrate the text and thank the ALSG/CAI Emergency Maternal and Child Health (EMCH) programme and the ALSG Managing Obstetric Emergencies and Trauma (MOET) course for the shared use of some of their line drawings.

Finally, we thank, in advance, those of you who will attend the POET course; no doubt, you will have much constructive critique to offer.

Contact details and website information

Advanced
Life
Support
Group

ALSG: www.alsg.org
BestBETS: www.bestbets.org

For details on ALSG courses visit the website or contact:
Advanced Life Support Group
ALSG Centre for Training and Development
29–31 Ellesmere Street
Swinton, Manchester
M27 0LA
Tel: +44 (0) 161 794 1999
Fax: +44 (0) 161 794 9111
Email: enquiries@alsg.org

Updates
The material contained within this book is updated on approximately a four-yearly cycle. However, practise may change in the interim period. We will post any changes on the ALSG website, so we advise you to visit the website regularly to check for updates (url: www.alsg.org – updates are on the course pages). The website will provide you with a new page to download and replace the existing page in your book.

References
To access references visit the ALSG website www.alsg.org – references are on the course pages.

On-line feedback
It is important to ALSG that the contact with our providers continues after a course is completed. We now contact everyone 6 months after his or her course has taken place asking for on-line feedback on the course. This information is then used whenever the course is updated to ensure that the course provides optimum training to its participants.

CHAPTER 1
Obstetric services

OBJECTIVES

Having read this chapter, the practitioner should be able to:
- understand the relationship between the different professional groups involved in the management of the obstetric patient
- understand the function and importance of hand-held records and how to use them effectively

ORGANISATION OF OBSTETRIC SERVICES, EPIDEMIOLOGY OF OBSTETRICS AND GYNAECOLOGICAL EMERGENCIES AND ROLE OF THE AMBULANCE SERVICE, GENERAL PRACTITIONER AND MIDWIFE

The organisation

Obstetrics is a multidisciplinary specialty in which midwifery and medical staff work together to provide optimal care. The majority of care is performed in the out-of-hospital setting and by community midwives. Inpatient antenatal care is now uncommon and not usually for long periods. Similarly, the postnatal length of stay for all women, even those with Caesarean section, has also been reduced, with the majority of care occurring in the community.

General practitioners (GPs) have in recent years become less and less involved in all aspects of pregnancy care, although there are still a small number who are involved in care in labour.

Place of delivery

Women undergo a risk assessment prior to delivery to help them choose where to deliver. This assessment is undertaken by their

Pre-Hospital Obstetric Emergency Training, 1st edition. By Malcolm Woollard, Kim Hinshaw, Helen Simpson and Sue Wieteska. Published 2010 by Blackwell Publishing, ISBN: 978-1-4051-8475-5.

1

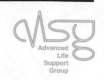

midwife in conjunction with medical staff, if required, and will involve assessment of previous medical history, previous obstetric history and the progress of the current pregnancy. They will then be offered advice to help them choose the place of birth.

A woman may choose to have a home delivery, deliver in a midwifery-led unit which may or may not be attached to a consultant-led unit or in a consultant-led unit. Although in the majority of cases women 'choose' the appropriate place to deliver, midwives have a duty of care to support the woman's final choice of place for delivery even if there are factors that make this a high-risk decision. Occasionally this causes difficulties, for example, in home delivery where access is poor, there is no phone signal or the home environment is less than ideal. Some women with a high-risk pregnancy also request home delivery.

Mode of delivery

The majority of deliveries are uncomplicated but the national Caesarean section rate is 23%. However, this rate varies significantly between units (range 15–30%). Caesarean section is major surgery and can have significant associated risks for both mother and baby.

Common 999 emergencies

- labour +/− delivery (term or preterm)
- bleeding antenatally or postnatally (including miscarriage) and postoperative gynaecological haemorrhage
- abdominal pain other than labour
- eclampsia (this is now less common, 2:10,000 cases due to the use of magnesium sulphate in hospital in at-risk cases; however, this does mean that one of the more common places to have a fit, will be in the community)
- prolapsed umbilical cord

Transfer

This occurs where risk factors develop before or during labour and after birth that necessitate moving the woman or baby from one location to another.

Transfer may be required from all places of delivery.

Transfer from home delivery

The commonest reasons for transfer are concerns about the progress of labour, fetal or maternal well-being, or neonatal well-being.

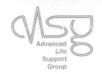

Transfer from midwifery-led unit

The commonest reasons for transfer are concerns about labour progress, fetal or maternal well-being, or neonatal well-being.

Transfer from a consultant-led unit

The commonest reason for transfer is the need to access a neonatal cot for the fetus either because the unit they are in does not have the appropriate neonatal facilities or all the cots are full. Occasionally women need to be moved to other units for maternal specialist care.

In all these scenarios, a midwife (or medical staff) will accompany the women and will be an invaluable source of advice and knowledge if problems occur during transfer. See Table 1.1 for the roles undertaken by clinical staff.

Top tip

If delivery is imminent, divert to the nearest unit rather than the planned unit.

Table 1.1 Roles of medical staff.

	Paramedic	Midwife	GP (if on scene)	Obstetrician (via telephone)
Clinical condition	Assess	Assess	Assess	
Initiate holding treatment	ALS Obstetric support	Assist with ALS Obstetric expertise	Assist with ALS Obstetric support*	Advice on treatment
Transfer	Provide transportation Liaise with receiving unit Confirm exact location of receiving obstetric unit within hospital	Advice on most appropriate receiving unit Liaise with receiving unit Advice on timing/need for transfer		Advice on most appropriate receiving unit Liaise with referring crew Advice on timing/need for transfer
Advice		Obstetric expertise	General issues	Obstetric expertise

*Some GPs have specific expertise in obstetrics.

Roles

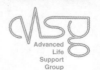

> **Top tip**
>
> Many features of the clinical management of an obstetric patient during secondary transfer are similar to that required in the home or during primary hospital admission. For example, remember to transport the patient in the 15–30° left lateral tilt position.

> **Top tip**
>
> Scoop and run is often the way forward with obstetric emergencies.

Further information on the management of inter-hospital transfers generally and neonatal transfers specifically can be found in the STaR (P. Driscoll et al. 2006) and PaNSTaR (S. Byrne et al. 2008) textbooks respectively.

Admissions procedures

These depend on local policies. Obstetric patients are usually admitted directly to the maternity unit, such as a triage or assessment unit or labour ward. In the case of major trauma, obstetric patients should be transferred to the emergency department. In the case of medical problems admit via medical pathways.

In many units, cases with early pregnancy problems will be admitted to the gynaecology department via an early pregnancy assessment unit.

USING PATIENT HAND-HELD RECORDS

Most maternity units in the UK provide women with their own maternity hand-held notes (see Fig. 1.1). Women are reported to feel better informed by holding responsibility for these notes, and are more involved in their maternity care. Carrying these notes also gives them increased satisfaction in the promotion of communication between themselves and health care providers (DH 2006).

Many instances of adverse perinatal and maternal mortality and morbidity are potentially avoidable, and are often linked to a lack of communication (Elbourne et al. 1987). The hand-held maternity notes are, therefore, an important link for health care providers to improve care and reduce error.

MATERNITY UNIT

MATERNITY NOTES OF:

NAME:
ADDRESS:
TELEPHONE:
DATE OF BIRTH:
HOSPITAL NO:

NAMED MIDWIFE

TEAM

CONSULTANT   USS EDD:-

GP   GP TEL NOS.

AMBULANCE NUMBER:

PLEASE CARRY THESE NOTES WITH YOU AT ALL TIMES

Figure 1.1 Example front cover of Patient hand-held records.

Although there is widespread variation in maternity hand-held notes throughout the UK, the general principles apply throughout:
• The front cover will display the woman's name, address, named midwife, consultant and GP.
• Information within the notes for the woman to read, including appropriate advice line numbers, screening tests and routine visits.
• The notes will identify whether the woman is on the low- or high-risk pathway of care. This is dependent on factors identified within this pregnancy or previous pregnancies and current medical condition.
• The antenatal section will display all screening tests performed, routine antenatal visits, scan results and fetal growth monitoring.
• There will be a section for the woman to complete a birth plan, in discussion with her midwife.

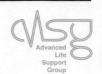

- There is a labour and postnatal section, which also includes detailed information regarding the baby, such as condition at delivery, findings on the neonatal examination and details on feeding.
- All investigations and screening tests will be reported.
- **Most hand-held notes have an alert page or box**. This will identify any complications or potential complications, and may show a plan of care to address these complications. **Any health professional can and should annotate this page**.
- There will be a section for correspondence between health care professionals, identifying potential problems and formulating plans of care. **Any health professional can and should annotate this page**.
- Ambulance crews attending an obstetric patient who has not been transported to hospital should leave a copy of their patient report form in the hand-held records.

It is paramount that the hand-held notes accompany the woman for all hospital admissions and routine antenatal visits. However, the notes may not have been issued to a woman in very early pregnancy if she has not booked through her midwife. It is still worth checking with her.

SUMMARY OF KEY POINTS

It is important that you are aware of the roles of other health care professionals in the care of the obstetric patient. Remember that any health professional can and should annotate the alert page in the patient's hand-held notes.

CHAPTER 2

Law, ethics and governance related to pregnancy

OBJECTIVES

Having read this chapter, the practitioner should be able to:
- discuss the impact of obstetric-related incidents on litigation claims made against UK ambulance services
- describe the process of gaining consent from adult patients and minors
- discuss the importance of maintaining patient confidentiality and the legal context for this
- debate the appropriateness of pronouncing death in obstetric cases
- state the common causes of complaints
- define negligence and describe the components necessary to demonstrate its proof
- discuss the impact of varied cultural issues on the provision of obstetric care in the pre-hospital setting
- state the professional responsibilities of pre-hospital practitioners
- describe the process of medicines management in the pre-hospital setting
- discuss the role of the employer and the employee with respect to the Health and Safety at Work Act 1974

INTRODUCTION

A significant proportion of the more costly litigation claims made against UK ambulance services arise from pre-hospital obstetric incidents. Although in a 10-year period, obstetric cases consisted of only 13 of the total 272 claims, the average value of these cases was £815,000. Four were valued at more than £1 million. Claims were based on either an alleged failure to identify and manage a problem or a lack of appropriate equipment for the treatment of a

---

Pre-Hospital Obstetric Emergency Training, 1st edition. By Malcolm Woollard, Kim Hinshaw, Helen Simpson and Sue Wieteska. Published 2010 by Blackwell Publishing, ISBN: 978-1-4051-8475-5.

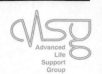

preterm baby. The largest claim was for £3,375,000 and related to an alleged lack of equipment to care for a baby born at 26 weeks (Dobbie and Cooke 2008).

Although the numbers of women and babies dying as a result of obstetric emergencies in the UK are small, some of these deaths might be prevented if effective training in the prompt recognition and management of these cases is undertaken by pre-hospital providers (Woollard et al. 2008). Although it could be argued that antenatal provision of preventive obstetric care is more effective than treating problems after they arise, the Confidential Enquiry into Maternal and Child Health (CEMACH) report suggests that many of the pregnant women who died *'had chaotic lifestyles and found it hard to engage with maternity services'*. One of its 'top ten' recommendations states:

> All clinical staff must undertake regular, written, documented and audited training for:
> - The identification, initial management and referral for serious medical and mental health conditions which, although unrelated to pregnancy, may affect pregnant women or recently delivered mothers
> - The early recognition and management of severely ill pregnant women and impending maternal collapse
> - The improvement of basic, immediate and advanced life support skills. A number of courses provide additional training for staff caring for pregnant women and newborn babies.
> There is also a need for staff to recognise their limitations and to know when, how and whom to call for assistance.
> (CEMACH 2007c)

In 1999, a new obstetrics and gynaecology section was added to the paramedic manual and became a mandatory part of the course, and subsequently part of the requirements for paramedic registration (Dawson et al. 1999). It was expected that these materials would be taught to student paramedics over five days, and that paramedics who had already qualified in earlier years, would receive update training as a component of their mandatory three-yearly re-qualification classes. Anecdotal reports suggest, however, that these educational aspirations are often not met, with training sessions being limited in duration and often not being delivered by practicing obstetricians and midwives.

All registered health care professionals are ultimately responsible for their own competence, and this extends to identifying their own training needs and taking steps to ensure these are met. A strong motivation for doing so, other than the obvious one of being able to meet patient's needs, is individual accountability for practice. A failure to provide acceptable standards of care, not only risks the patient's welfare but also the practitioner's registration and ability to earn a living in their chosen career. Although obstetric emergencies are rare, the consequences of mishandling them can be particularly severe for mother and baby, and also for the pre-hospital practitioner.

CONSENT

Although it is incumbent upon all health care providers to practise only in the interests of their patients, this principle is sometimes misunderstood by paternalistic practitioners as overriding the wishes of the patient themselves. However, the need to obtain consent before providing treatment is paramount: all *competent* adults have an inherent right to self-determination, even if their wishes may result in harm to themselves. Significantly, in UK obstetric practice, the fetus itself has no legal rights independent of the mother until after delivery has occurred. One example is a mother who declines delivery by emergency Caesarean section when there is obvious evidence of potential hypoxia affecting the fetus in labour. If she is deemed to be *competent* in terms of making that decision, to enforce the operation would likely be viewed as an assault under criminal law.

Consent should, wherever possible, be provided on an informed basis. This requires that the patient not only understands what precise intervention is proposed, but has also been advised of the potential benefits and possible adverse effects of the treatment, and of the relative advantages and disadvantages of alternative therapeutic options. They must also understand that they can decline/refuse proposed treatment if they wish, but should be fully informed of the potential consequences of doing so, to themselves and their baby. Failure to fully explain to a patient what might go wrong if they do not receive the proposed care risks a charge of professional negligence. In these circumstances, it is critically important that the discussions should be carefully documented in detail in clinical records. Patients who decline/refuse treatment (or a recommendation for admission to hospital) should always be advised that they can call for further help at any time, and should be informed about any symptoms that might indicate their condition is deteriorating. Remember, administering treatment to a competent adult against their will exposes the practitioner to the possibility of being prosecuted for assault under criminal law. Simply 'threatening' to provide treatment against a person's wishes could be judged as assault in common law.

Patients may demonstrate consent in a number of ways: all are considered to be equally valid in the eyes of the law, and consent does not need to be confirmed in writing by the patient. Health care providers must, on the other hand, document in clinical records that consent has been obtained. Express consent is obtained if a patient specifically grants permission for a particular treatment to be carried out. For example, the practitioner may describe a proposed procedure in detail after which the patient verbally agrees to the intervention. Consent may also be *implied* – for example, a practitioner may explain to the patient that they wish to give them an injection of a pain-killing drug. If the patient offers their arm to the practitioner, consent has been implied. *Presumed* consent may only be inferred in cases where the patient is not able to give consent, either because they lack competency or because they are unconscious, *and* the treatment is necessary to save a life or prevent deterioration (the doctrine of necessity). This means that the practitioner is deemed to be acting 'in the patient's best interest'. Treatment of a less urgent nature may *not* be given using this principle.

In modern obstetric care, practitioners are sometimes required to provide treatment to patients who are legally minors (aged less than 18 years). Patients aged 16 years and over should be treated as competent adults and informed consent sought in the same way. This is also true for those aged less than 16 years, if it can be demonstrated that they have sufficient understanding and intelligence to enable them to comprehend fully what is proposed (sometimes referred to as 'Gillick competence' or 'Fraser guidelines'). In both cases someone with parental responsibility cannot overrule the wishes of a minor consenting to treatment. However, they *can* overrule a minor's decision to decline life-saving treatment as it can reasonably be argued that the patient is not sufficiently competent to understand the need for care. In the case of minors who are not competent to make decisions about their care, consent can be obtained from someone with parental responsibility for the child. If no such person is immediately available, the doctrine of necessity can be invoked to provide life-saving treatment. If a person with parental responsibility refuses life-saving treatment for the minor, a court order should ideally be obtained. However, if time does not permit a full explanation to be given to the parent, the intervention will need to be provided and the necessity of the treatment must be *witnessed* and *documented* (that is, the need for the specific treatment should be confirmed in writing in the clinical records by a colleague). In such circumstances, practitioners should contact their defence organisation as soon as possible after the incident (Fig. 2.1).

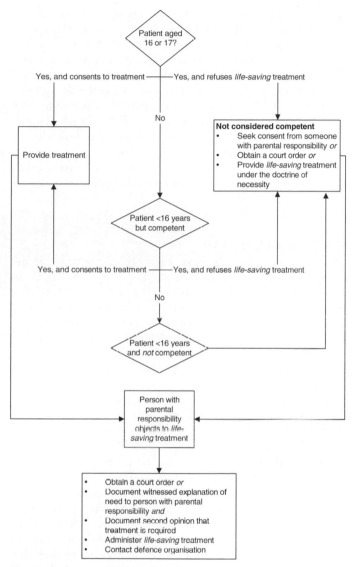

Figure 2.1 Consent process for minors.

CONFIDENTIALITY

All health care practitioners have a duty of confidentiality to their patients. This is espoused in codes of conduct issued by relevant professional bodies such as the Health Professions Council, the Nursing and Midwifery Council and the General Medical Council. It is also a requirement placed on employees by all NHS trusts.

However, patient's confidentiality is also protected in law by the Data Protection Act (1998), and it should be noted that this applies equally to all forms of records, not just those stored on computer media. Practitioners must ensure that any information is only used for the purposes for which it was originally collected. They must take particular care to ensure that patient identifiable and clinical information is only shared with other health care providers with responsibility for care of the patient. This applies even when handing over in the emergency department or obstetric unit – never verbally present such information in the presence of relatives – either of the patient concerned or of anyone else. Be particularly careful in the pre-hospital setting when passing information to colleagues via telephone or radio.

PRONOUNCING DEATH

In recent years, protocols have been developed that permit pre-hospital practitioners, including paramedics and nurses, to pronounce death in certain circumstances in the out-of-hospital setting without the need to refer to a doctor. Nevertheless, practitioners should generally not pronounce death or terminate resuscitation in pregnant women unless the death is non-recent, as even if resuscitation of the mother is futile in rare cases the fetus may be saved. Similarly, in the absence of gross deformities incompatible with life, practitioners should initiate and continue resuscitation attempts for babies that have no signs of life after delivery until handover to emergency department staff.

MEDICAL ERRORS AND NEGLIGENCE

All serious untoward events or *potential* serious untoward events ('near-misses') should be reported in accordance with the employer's policy for incident reporting. It is NHS policy that genuine errors (as opposed to deliberate acts of negligence or non-conformance with documented procedures) should be investigated in a manner consistent with a 'no-blame' culture. This ensures that lessons can be learned from mistakes and changes made to training, policy or systems to avoid them being repeated. Measures are in place to facilitate lessons learned at NHS trust level being shared nationally, and this forms an important part of quality control in the UK health service.

The significant majority of formal complaints made against staff in the NHS are associated with the patient's or relative's perception that a practitioner had an unhelpful or aggressive attitude (Health

Care Commission, personal communication). A wise doctrine to remember is that *'Bad doctors get sued, and good doctors get sued, but nice doctors* don't *get sued'* (J. Clawson, personal communication). All health care practitioners are regularly required to deal with situations or people that they consider unpleasant or difficult. It is inevitable that we make personal judgements in such circumstances: after all, we are only human. However, it is vital that such personal perceptions are not permitted to affect how we relate to the patient or their relatives and friends, and should never have any part to play in reaching clinical decisions. Such views should be kept to one's self, and no one external to the practitioner should be permitted the opportunity to perceive them. If a practitioner inadvertently offends someone, they should use the highly effective strategy of apologising. However, practitioners should not admit to making a clinical error without first taking further advice.

In the event of a complaint being received, the NHS has standards for how trusts should handle them, and in particular the time scale within which a response should be provided and the appeals process which should be made available to the complainant should they be unhappy with the response.

As has been implied previously, pre-hospital practitioners are at risk of being taken to court for alleged negligence. A negligent practitioner is one who has:

> Failed to exercise that degree of care which a person of ordinary prudence with the same or similar training would exercise in the same or similar circumstances. (Woollard and Todd 2006)

The case of *Bolam v. Friern Hospital Management Committee* (1957) established the precedent that to avoid being considered negligent a practitioner should provide care to 'the standard of an ordinary man professing to have that special skill. . .'. Negligence claims may arise as a result of an alleged act of omission or commission, and require that each of four components is demonstrated – which is often difficult to achieve. The first component is the *duty* to act. By responding to a request for assistance in the pre-hospital setting the practitioner automatically assumes such a duty, and the same is true if they report for work in a role which requires them to respond to such requests. The second component is *breach of duty* – essentially the failure to act (for example, to respond to a call or to provide care) when one has an established duty to do so. The third feature that must be demonstrated is that *damage or harm has taken place*. The final component to prove is *causation* – it must be shown that the harm that the patient experienced was as a direct result of the practitioner's breach of duty. This can be very difficult to prove. For example, if a practitioner fails to provide a shock at an appropriate energy setting for a patient in ventricular fibrillation, it could be demonstrated that a breach of duty had occurred by comparing the standard of care that would be expected to have been provided by a similarly qualified provider. If the patient was not resuscitated and died, it could be shown that harm had taken place. However, since the patient was dead at the point the practitioner commenced care, it might be difficult to successfully argue that the failure to shock correctly caused the death (harm). On the other hand, an important aspect of assessing harm and causation is the concept of 'loss of opportunity'. This might occur in the context of obstetric care if a pre-hospital provider keeps a patient with a significant haemorrhage on scene for a protracted period of time to assess the effect of intravenous fluids, when in fact the patient requires urgent surgery. As a result of the delay of surgery which could definitively control the haemorrhage the patient might die, and they will have experienced a loss of opportunity to have life-saving treatment. Although in criminal law the standard of evidence which has to be achieved is 'proof beyond a reasonable doubt', this is not the case in civil law where the 'balance of probability' is assessed. This is actually calculated as a percentage: if it is more than 50%, it is likely that an act of negligence occurred, then the case will be found against the practitioner.

CULTURAL ISSUES

Pre-hospital providers should consider themselves as guests in their patient's homes (or lives). As such we should respect the cultural values of the patients we are asked to attend. We should not expect our patients to adhere to our personal values.

The UK is a multicultural society and all pre-hospital practitioners need a basic understanding of the range of value systems that they might encounter. In many communities it is not normal or acceptable for women to be examined by men, and this can be particularly difficult for patients in the context of gynaecological and obstetric emergencies. Wherever possible female practitioners should be tasked to care for such patients and circumstances may require that male providers are not present when intimate examinations or procedures take place. If male practitioners are tempted to take offence in such situations, they should remember that patients have the right of autonomy and self-determination and if such a compromise is necessary to obtain consent to treatment this is well within the patient's rights. If no female providers are

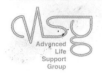

readily available in an emergency situation, male practitioners should explain the procedures that need to be carried out, and the consequences of delaying them, but ultimately a competent patient has the right to decline/refuse.

PROFESSIONAL ACCOUNTABILITY

Registered health care practitioners are personally accountable to their registrant body for the care that they provide to patients and have a number of responsibilities set out in their respective codes of conduct. These are similar across professional groups but the following list is taken from the Health Professions Council's Standards of Conduct, Performance and Ethics (Health Professions Council 2008):

1 You must act in the best interests of service users.
2 You must respect the confidentiality of service users.
3 You must keep high standards of personal conduct.
4 You must provide (to us and any other relevant regulators) any important information about your conduct and competence.
5 You must keep your professional knowledge and skills up to date.
6 You must act within the limits of your knowledge, skills and experience and, if necessary, refer the matter to another practitioner.
7 You must communicate properly and effectively with service users and other practitioners.
8 You must effectively supervise tasks that you have asked other people to carry out.
9 You must get informed consent to give treatment (except in an emergency).
10 You must keep accurate records.
11 You must deal fairly and safely with the risks of infection.
12 You must limit your work or stop practising if your performance or judgement is affected by your health.
13 You must behave with honesty and integrity and make sure that your behaviour does not damage the public's confidence in you or your profession.
14 You must make sure that any advertising you do is accurate.

MEDICINES MANAGEMENT

Doctors registered with the General Medical Council and nurses with a recognised qualification in Independent Prescribing that is recordable on their register may prescribe drugs within their competence. Paramedics are permitted to supply and administer prescription-only parenteral medicines that are listed for their specific use in the Medicines Act, and also those on the list of drugs that can be administered by anyone in an emergency. Both paramedics (and nurses without prescribing rights) may administer additional drugs on the basis of a patient group direction (PGD). These have a proscribed format, must be signed by the Chief Executive and Medical Director of the employing NHS trust and a senior pharmacist, and must list the practitioners authorised to use them. PGDs may not be used to authorise the use of controlled drugs, with the exception of midazolam.

There appears to be a common misconception that the standards for managing medicines, and even controlled drugs, in the pre-hospital setting are less rigorous than those in hospitals or are even waived. This is not the case. All prescription-only medicines must be accounted for and their use documented in each patient's records. Only those groups of practitioners with the appropriate rights as defined in law may be in possession of prescription-only medicines: for example, emergency medical technicians should not be in possession of drugs that are restricted by the Medicines Act to use by paramedics. Controlled drugs, such as opioids and benzodiazepines must be stored in a locked cabinet fixed to an immovable surface inside another locked cupboard or container. In the pre-hospital setting this requires vehicles to be fitted with a lockable drug safe bolted to the infrastructure inside the boot or another locked cupboard. Record keeping of controlled drugs must be as rigorous in pre-hospital care as it is in the hospital setting, and every ampoule must be accounted for and documented. Controlled drugs may be carried on the person of practitioners authorised in law to possess them. The failure to abide by the relevant legislation is a breach of criminal law and the consequences can be very severe.

HEALTH AND SAFETY AT WORK
It is the duty of employers under the Health and Safety at Work Act 1974 to take all reasonable precautions to minimise the risk to employees arising from their employment. This includes the provision of protective equipment, the formulation of policy and procedure, and provision of training. Importantly, the Act also places a duty on employees to utilise safety equipment provided to them by their employers, and to act in accordance with relevant policy and procedure. If an employee fails to do so and either they, a colleague, or a patient comes to harm as a result, that employee is in breach of the law.

Advanced
Life
Support
Group

SUMMARY OF KEY POINTS

- One of the most common subjects of high-cost litigation cases against UK ambulance services is obstetric care.
- The Confidential Enquiry into Maternal and Child Health has recommended that all practitioners with a responsibility for caring for obstetric patients receive training in the identification and management of obstetric emergencies.
- Informed consent must be sought from all adult competent patients before providing any treatment.
- Minors aged between 16 and 18 years and those younger than 16 years who are capable of understanding the proposed interventions may give consent to treatment. Such consent to treatment cannot be overruled, even by someone with parental responsibility. However, a person with parental responsibility can overrule a minor's decision not to have life-saving treatment.
- Practitioners have both a professional and legal duty to maintain patient confidentiality and only to use patient data for the purpose for which it was originally collated.
- In most circumstances, a pregnant woman should not be pronounced dead in the pre-hospital setting: resuscitation should be initiated and maintained even if the mother has no chance of survival as rarely the fetus may do so.
- Serious or potentially serious untoward events should be reported promptly through trust's established systems.
- A non-judgemental and friendly attitude to all patients will prevent most complaints being made.
- An appropriate apology can reduce the likelihood of a formal complaint.
- Negligence is the failure to act in accordance with the standards of an ordinary person with the same specialist skills.
- A duty to act, a breach of that duty, harm and causation must all be demonstrated with a greater than 50% probability for a negligence suit to be successful.
- All registered health practitioners are individually accountable for their own practice.
- Controlled drugs *cannot* be supplied and administered under a PGD.
- Controlled drug storage and documentation regulations are as robust in the pre-hospital setting as they are in-hospital.
- Both employers and employees have a legal responsibility for the safety of themselves, colleagues and patients under the Health and Safety at Work Act 1974.

CHAPTER 3

Anatomical and physiological changes in pregnancy

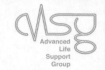

OBJECTIVES

Having read this chapter, the practitioner should be able to:
- describe the anatomical and physiological changes in the airway, breathing, circulatory, genital tract and gastrointestinal systems during pregnancy and their implications for management
- interpret common laboratory test results in pregnancy

ANATOMICAL AND PHYSIOLOGICAL CHANGES IN PREGNANCY AND IMPLICATIONS FOR MANAGEMENT

Airway

Although the airway itself does not change dramatically as a result of pregnancy, other anatomical and physiological changes will result in the need to modify priorities and strategies for airway management. Increasing numbers of pregnant women are morbidly obese, and this creates further management issues with the airway (Heslehurst et al. 2007). More than half of all the women who died from direct or indirect causes were either overweight or obese, of these more than 15% were morbidly or super morbidly obese (CEMACH 2007c).

The neck may appear short and obese, and the pregnant woman is likely to have engorged breasts, particularly in late pregnancy. If the patient is suffering from a hypertensive disorder, oedema of the upper airway may be present. Pregnant patients tend to be young and therefore are likely to have full dentition.

Pre-Hospital Obstetric Emergency Training, 1st edition. By Malcolm Woollard, Kim Hinshaw, Helen Simpson and Sue Wieteska. Published 2010 by Blackwell Publishing, ISBN: 978-1-4051-8475-5.

Physiological changes in the gastrointestinal system can also have significant implications for airway management. In the patient with a reduced conscious level, the risk of regurgitation, aspiration and Mendelson's syndrome increases due to a combination of factors:

- a relaxed gastro-oesophageal sphincter
- increased intragastric pressure
- delayed gastric emptying due to upward pressure on the diaphragm from the gravid uterus (again, particularly in the third trimester)

Top tip

Early intubation is essential in the pregnant patient without a gag reflex.

Breathing

In late pregnancy the tidal volume increases by 20% at 12 weeks and by 40% at 40 weeks. Because the total lung capacity is unchanged, this increase in tidal volume is at the expense of a proportionate decrease in inspiratory and expiratory reserve and residual capacity. Therefore, the patient will have a reduced ability to compensate for any increase in oxygen demand due to illness or injury.

Indeed, the normal physiological demands of pregnancy result in an increase in oxygen demand of 15% in the well pregnant patient. This is met by a small increase in respiratory rate as well as the increased tidal volume.

The shape of the rib cage changes, splaying out at its base due to the need to accommodate a gravid uterus. This reduces costal excursion and so the diaphragm plays an increasingly significant role in supporting respiration as the pregnancy progresses.

Top tip

Pregnant women have little respiratory reserve. Monitor oxygen saturation and give oxygen immediately if saturation on air falls below 94%. If SpO_2 is less than 85% use non-rebreathing mask; otherwise use a simple face mask. Aim for a target saturation of 94–98%.

Circulation

Blood volume rises throughout pregnancy, and by the last trimester it will have increased by 50%. Red cell numbers also rise, but since this is to a lesser degree than plasma volumes the actual haemoglobin concentration falls. This results in haemodilution compared to the non-pregnant state.

By the middle of pregnancy, cardiac output rises by approximately 40% due largely to an increase in the stroke volume. This is also due to a lesser extent, to an increase in the pulse rate to about 85–100 at the end of the third trimester. However, the workload of the heart is not increased due to the reduction in blood viscosity (as a result of haemodilution) and decreased peripheral vascular resistance (reduced afterload).

> **Top tip**
>
> **Extrasystoles are common in pregnancy and are usually harmless.**

Cardiac output increases due to:
- hormone-mediated peripheral vasodilation
- greater metabolic requirements arising from increased organ size and activity (particularly relating to the lungs, kidneys, gastrointestinal system and skin)
- increased heat production (resulting in vasodilation in the skin)
- the placenta's function as a shunt between the arterial and venous systems (the lack of a capillary system where branches of the uterine artery connect directly to the placental venous sinuses results in a lowered peripheral resistance)

The reduction in peripheral vascular resistance places pregnant women at risk of postural hypotension due to the potential for a sudden drop in systolic blood pressure when moving to a standing position. This may result in cerebral hypoperfusion and consequently syncope. To avoid this risk, pregnant women should be encouraged to move from a lying to a sitting or sitting to standing position slowly – for example, if they are moving from lying to standing they should:
- sit up with legs out straight
- wait for a few seconds then check for dizziness
- move so that their legs are dependent over the edge of the bed
- wait for a few seconds then check for dizziness
- stand up

At the beginning of pregnancy the systolic blood pressure falls, but returns to near normal levels at term. Despite this the pulse pressure increases due to a relatively greater fall in diastolic pressure. As in all patients, the systolic blood pressure provides a more useful indicator of patient status than the diastolic, with the exception that the diastolic is as important as systolic pressure in hypertension. The diastolic pressure should be documented at the point the sounds disappear (Korotkoff V). Occasionally in pregnancy, the sounds may not disappear. In that circumstance, diastolic BP can be estimated by noting when the sounds become muffled (Korotkoff IV).

Varicose veins often occur in the legs due to an increase in venous pressure, the relaxation of smooth muscle of the veins due to the effects of progesterone, and the presence of peripheral oedema.

During the late second and third trimester of pregnancy, if the patient lays flat on her back, the gravid uterus can result in supine hypotension due to aortocaval compression. The weight of the uterus compresses the inferior vena cava reducing venous return, in turn reducing cardiac filling and causing a fall in cardiac output. In response, arterial vasoconstriction occurs but arterial pressure will nevertheless fall if vena caval compression is not rapidly corrected, and the resulting low intra-aortic pressure will allow the aorta to be compressed. The effect on the patient is maternal syncope due to reduced cerebral perfusion and fetal hypoxia due to uterine hypoperfusion: in pre-existing low output states such as hypovolaemic shock or chest compressions during cardiac arrest the net result may be little or no maternal and fetal circulation.

Top tip

Women in the third trimester of pregnancy should NEVER be laid flat on their back. Always place a pillow underneath the right buttock. This will not be adequate in a morbidly obese patient: it may be necessary to use a spine board tilted at 15–30°.

Top tip

If the patient is obtunded, the easiest way to tip the patient to their left is to strap them to a spine board and place pillows or folded blankets under the board to provide a 15–30° tilt. This provides a solid surface against which to perform chest compressions if necessary (see Fig. 3.1).

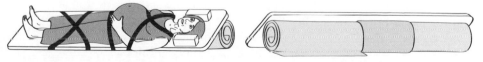

View from behind. Tilt 15–30°

(a)   (b)

Figure 3.1 Spineboard.

Top tip

If CPR is **unlikely** to be required, place the patient in the 15–30° or full left lateral position.

Top tip

Most ambulances receive patients on stretchers 'head first'. If the patient is in the 15–30° left lateral position they will be facing the wall of the saloon. Either load the patient feet first, or if this is not possible, ensure you check their airway continuously.

The important thing is transporting the patient safely: this may mean moving her into the right lateral position.

Top tip

In an emergency, the uterus can be lifted and manually displaced to the left provided sufficient personnel are present (see Fig. 3.2).

In the event of hypovolaemic shock, the normal physiological changes of pregnancy (increased plasma and red cell volume) allow the patient to compensate for some time. This can make diagnosis difficult as changes in vital signs may be minimal: instead the practitioner must rely on identifying external blood loss or by having a high index of suspicion for internal concealed haemorrhage.

The main mechanism of maintaining maternal circulation in the event of blood loss is the restriction of blood flow to the uterus. This can occur rapidly following the onset of significant bleeding, and will result in a reduction in placental perfusion with associated fetal hypoxia. Consequently even in the absence of signs of shock, control of haemorrhage and restoration of circulating volume have the highest priority.

If blood loss continues there are few other compensatory mechanisms remaining, since stroke volume is already increased as a normal physiological change of pregnancy. Although the heart rate may rise, this has only a minimal effect. At this point, the patient is likely to decompensate rapidly, and this is very difficult to reverse. Consequently rapid diagnosis and transportation to a hospital with obstetric surgical facilities (with a pre-alert on route) is

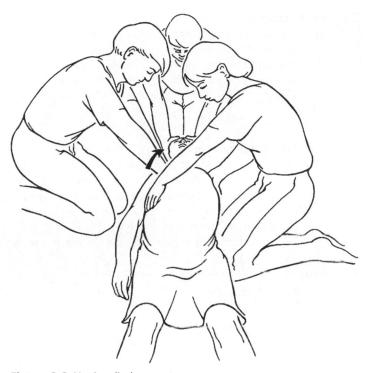

Figure 3.2 Uterine displacement.

essential to facilitate control of haemorrhage at the earliest possible time. Cannulation and intravenous fluids should only be initiated on route to hospital to avoid any delay on scene.

Top tip

Delaying on scene to start an intravenous infusion only allows further blood loss to occur and greatly increases the risk of irreversible decompensation.

Top tip

The treatment of obstetric haemorrhage is early surgery. This is best facilitated by short on-scene times and a pre alert message to the hospital.

The genital tract

The uterus and genital tract enlarge during pregnancy and the blood supply increases to meet the energy requirements of the muscular uterus and the growing fetus. The high muscle tone in the uterus raises the risk of it tearing following trauma, and its excellent blood supply significantly increases the likelihood of major haemorrhage.

The gastrointestinal system

As described in the airway section, gastric tone and emptying rates are reduced in pregnancy, particularly during late pregnancy and even more so during labour. Although secretion of gastric acid is reduced in mid-pregnancy this rises above normal levels at the end of the third trimester. The cardiac sphincter is relatively lax as a consequence of the effects of progesterone, and the gravid uterus compresses the stomach, potentially displacing its contents into the oesophagus. As a consequence of these changes, there is a greater risk of gastric reflux and aspiration, made worse by the increased acidity of stomach contents.

Top tip

Failure to effectively secure the airway in unconscious pregnant patients is associated with an increased risk of aspiration pneumonia.

RELEVANT LABORATORY TESTS – DIFFERENCES IN THE 'NORMAL RANGE' IN PREGNANCY

Table 3.1 shows the main differences in results between the pregnant and non-pregnant state (Heslehurst et al. 2007). When no difference occurs then the non-pregnant value is given. Table 3.2 provides a summary of key points.

Some tests vary according to gestation in which cases the range of values covers all stages.

Table 3.3 gives examples of blood results obtained in different clinical conditions (this is not an exhaustive list but contains some common or important examples).

Table 3.1 Ranges of values for laboratory tests.

Test	Non-pregnant	Pregnant/ immediate postnatal	Reason
Full blood count			
Hb (g/dl)	12–15	11–14	Haemodilution
WBC × 10^9 per litre	4–11	6–16	Due to increased neutrophil count
Platelets × 10^9 per litre	150–400		
MCV (fl)	80–100		
CRP (g/l)	0–7		
Renal function			
Urea (mmol/l)	2.5–7.5	2.4–4.2	Increase in GFR Vasodilatation
Creatinine (micromol/l)	65–101	44–73	Lowest in mid-trimester
K (mmol/l)	3.5–5.0	3.3–4.1	
Na (mmol/l)	135–145	130–140	
Uric acid (mmol/l)	0.18–0.35	0.14–0.38	
24-hour protein (g)	<0.15	<0.3	
24-hour creatinine	70–140	119–169	
Bilirubin (micromol/l)	0–17	3–16	
Total protein (g/l)	64–86	48–64	
Albumin (g/l)	35–46	28–37	
AST (IU/l)	7–40	10 30	
ALT (IU/l)	0–40	6–32	
GGT (IU/l)	11–50	3–43	
Alk Phos (IU/l)	30–130	32–418	Produced by placenta; highest in third trimester
Bile acids (micromol/l)	0–17		
TFTs			
fT4 (pmol/l)	11–23	10.6–20.4	
fT3 (pmol/l)	4–9	3.4–7.1	
TSH (mu/l)	0–4	0.09–3.03	

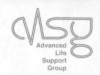

Table 3.2 Summary of key points.

Lower in pregnancy	Higher in pregnancy
Haemoglobin	White cell count
Urea	Alk Phos
Creatinine	pH
Sodium	PaO_2
Potassium	
Protein	
Albumin	
Bilirubin	
AST	
ALT	
Gamma GT	
Free T4	
Free T3	
Bicarbonate	
$PaCO_2$	

Table 3.3 Interpretation of abnormal values.

Test	High	Low
Haemoglobin		Anaemia
		Sickle-cell disease
		Thalassaemia
White cell count	Infection	
Clotting factors		DIC
(APPT, PT)		Abruption
		Severe pre-eclampsia
Urea and creatinine	Renal failure	
	Dehydration	
	Pre-eclampsia	
Urate	Pre-eclampsia	
Total protein/albumin		Renal failure
		Pre-eclampsia
Liver function tests	Severe pre-eclampsia	
	HELLP	
	Cholestasis	
	Hepatitis (viral)	
	Acute fatty liver of	
	pregnancy	
Platelets		Severe pre-eclampsia
		HELLP
		DIC
Glucose	Diabetes	Acute fatty liver of
		pregnancy

SUMMARY OF KEY POINTS

- Early definitive airway management is essential in any obtunded obstetric patient as changes to the GI system increase the risk of aspiration.
- Pregnant patients have little respiratory reserve.
- Pregnant patients may initially compensate for blood loss due to their increased circulatory volume; however, this will be at the expense of the blood supply to the fetus.
- Pregnant patients may suddenly decompensate rapidly following haemorrhage: this is often irreversible.
- Pregnant women are at increased risk of postural hypotension and should be encouraged to change position slowly.
- Never lie a patient in the late second or third trimester supine to avoid vena caval compression, which can lead to maternal and fetal hypoxia.

CHAPTER 4
Normal delivery

OBJECTIVES

Having read this chapter, the practitioner should be able to:
- understand the mechanism of normal delivery

NORMAL LABOUR AND DELIVERY

The anatomy of the female pelvis (Fig. 4.1)

Pelvic inlet

This is the superior margin of the pelvis and is bounded by the sacral promontory posteriorly, laterally by the iliopectineal lines and anteriorly by the symphysis. It tends to be larger in the transverse diameter than in the AP (anterior/posterior) diameter.

Pelvic cavity

This is bounded by the symphysis pubis anteriorly, laterally by the pubic bone and the obturator fascia and the inner aspect of the ischial bone and posteriorly by the sacrum. The transverse and AP diameter tend to be similar

Pelvic outlet

This is the inferior margin of the pelvis. This is bounded posteriorly by the coccyx, laterally by the ischial tuberosities and anteriorly

---

Pre-Hospital Obstetric Emergency Training, 1st edition. By Malcolm Woollard, Kim Hinshaw, Helen Simpson and Sue Wieteska. Published 2010 by Blackwell Publishing, ISBN: 978-1-4051-8475-5.

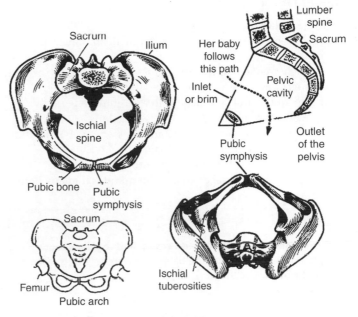

Figure 4.1 Anatomy of the female pelvis.

by the pubic arch. The AP diameter tends to be bigger than the transverse diameter.

Anatomy of the fetal skull

The fetal skull can be divided into the vault, face and base. At birth the bones of the vault are not united allowing moulding to occur (see Fig. 4.2).

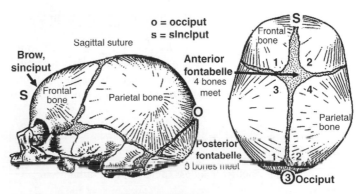

Figure 4.2 Anatomy of the fetal skull.

Stages of labour

First stage of labour

- Defined as contractions causing cervical dilatation from 0 to 10 cm.
- Increasingly frequent and more regular contractions as the first stage progresses.
- Count the number of contractions in a 10-minute period.
- In established labour, there are 3–4 contractions in 10 minutes.
- More than five contractions in 10 minutes are overstimulation and may suggest abruption (see Chapter 7).
- Contractions can last for about 1 minute.
- The length of the first stage can be from minutes to many hours.

> **Top tip**
>
> At 8 cm, women are often very distressed and regularly request an epidural or demand that the baby is delivered – this is often one of the most vocal stages.

> **Top tip**
>
> Labour is often faster in second and subsequent pregnancies.

Precipitant labour

This is a very fast labour with a duration of less than 1 hour.

Membranes

- These can rupture at any point before or during labour.
- Liquor should be clear and odourless.
- If liquor is blood stained, this could indicate an abruption or placenta praevia.
- If liquor is meconium stained (yellow- or green-coloured liquor which can be thin and watery or thick with particulate material), this can be an indicator of fetal compromise and it should be noted that the presence of particulate material is a particular cause for concern (see Chapter 9).

> **Top tip**
>
> Always consider whether fluid loss could be urine rather than liquor.

Second stage

- It occurs once fully dilated (10 cm).
- Women may have a strong urge to push, this may be a very similar feeling to opening bowels and may often result in the bowels being opened.
- The vertex may be visible at the introitus. In the situation where no midwife is present, this will be the only way of confirming the second stage.
- Second stage is completed by delivery of the baby (see below for the mechanism of normal delivery).

Top tip

Occasionally membranes will be visible at the vaginal entrance but the presenting part will be much higher and the cervix may not be fully dilated.

Third stage

- This begins with the delivery of the baby and is complete with delivery of the placenta.
- If the placenta stays in situ for more than 30 minutes after an active second stage, it is considered to be retained. A period of 60 minutes can be allowed if a physiological second stage (that is without the use of drugs or controlled cord traction) has occurred.
- If the placenta partially separates, bleeding can be torrential and urgent action is required – see chapter on postpartum haemorrhage (Chapter 8).

The normal mechanism of labour

- The mechanism of labour is the passive way in which the fetus makes its way through the birth canal.
- The movements allow the fetus to negotiate the changing dimensions of the pelvis.
- The widest diameter of the pelvic brim is the transverse dimension, whereas the widest diameter of the outlet is the AP (anterior/posterior dimension). Thus the widest part of the fetal head enters the pelvis in the transverse dimension and then rotates to emerge in the AP diameter at the outlet.
- The shoulders similarly follow the rotation.
- The commonest presentation is the vertex and the commonest positions are either left or right occipitoanterior. The lie will be longitudinal and the attitude one of flexion. The engaging diameter of the fetal head is therefore the suboccipitobregmatic.

Descent
Descent often starts before labour, as the fetal head becomes engaged in the pelvis. In the multigravid woman engagement may not occur until labour commences. Further descent through the pelvis occurs during labour.

Flexion
When labour starts the head will be in a position of natural flexion. This is increased during labour for two reasons:
- Any ovoid object being passed through a tube tends to adapt its long axis to the long axis of the tube.
- Head lever – the occipitospinal joint is nearer to the occiput than the sinciput. When the uterus contracts and pressure is applied to the fetal breech the direction of push naturally flexes the head.

Internal rotation (Fig. 4.3)
As labour continues the fetal head meets the resistance of the pelvic floor and the occiput rotates forwards from the occipitotransverse or occipitoanterior position to lie under the suprapubic arch, with the sagittal suture lying in the AP diameter. The rotation occurs because, in addition to the well-flexed head, the sloping gutter shape of the levatores ani (pelvic muscles) directs the occiput (which is leading) anteriorly.

The head will then appear at the introitus. The accoucheur can control head delivery by gentle pressure.

Crowning
The fetal head has crowned when it emerges from under the pubic arch and no longer recedes between contractions. It will be visible at the introitus.

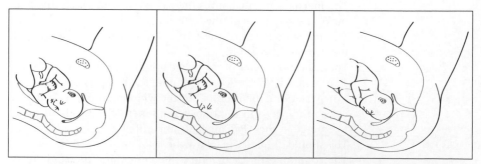

Head enters the pelvic brim   As head descends the back of   The head is in the lower pelvis
                               the head usually rotates to the front   and has rotated to the front

Figure 4.3 Diagram of internal rotation.

Encouraging the woman to pant/breathe through the contraction at this stage will help control the delivery of the head.

Extension
The head then delivers by extension. Once the occiput has passed below the symphysis pubis, the head extends with the nape of the neck pressed firmly against the pubic arch. As extension continues the forehead, face and chin deliver over the perineum. It is not necessary to check for cord as usually the body will deliver through any loops of cord: the need to cut and divide is rare.

Restitution
As internal rotation occurs the fetal head becomes twisted a little on the shoulders. As soon as it is delivered it resumes its natural position, with respect to the shoulders. This is called restitution.

External rotation (Fig. 4.4)
At delivery of the head the shoulders lie in the oblique. With continued descent they rotate to bring the bisacromial diameter into

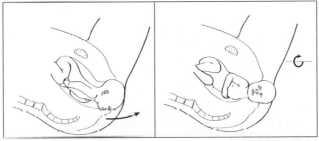

1. As the mother pushes, the head delivers by anteriorly ('upwards' with woman on her back)

2. After the head has delivered, the shoulders and head 'restitute' (i.e. they rotate 90° so head lies transversely again)

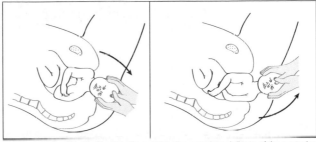

3. The anterior (front) shoulder then delivers when the mother pushes. Guide head **gently** downwards as she pushes until shoulder delivers

4. Finally, complete delivery of the posterior shoulder by **gentle** traction upwards. The body will follow after the shoulder. Deliver baby onto mother's abdomen

Figure 4.4 Diagram of external rotation.

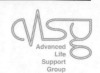

the AP diameter of the pelvic outlet. Rotation of the shoulders occurs as the right and anterior shoulder is lower than the left in the pelvis and meets the resistance of the pelvic floor before the left, it therefore rotates to the space in the front. This causes the head to rotate so that the occiput lies next to the maternal left thigh. This is external rotation. If the fetus is lying the other way around this description should be reversed.

Delivery of the body

The anterior shoulder is now able to pass under the pubis and with lateral flexion of the body the posterior arm is born. The rest of the body follows easily. If necessary gently guide the body downwards initially then as the anterior shoulder is delivered lift the baby upwards.

Pass the baby up to the mother and ensure skin-to-skin contact to maintain warmth, or resuscitate as necessary.

Top tip

Most babies, if left to their own devices, will deliver spontaneously without any assistance.

Top tip

Pulling too hard on the baby at delivery can cause a brachial plexus injury.

Cutting the cord

Wait for the cord to stop pulsating before cutting and dividing unless the baby requires resuscitation.

To clamp the cord, place one cord clamp 1–2 cm from the baby's abdomen and a second clamp 2–3 cm distally to the first. Ensure that they are firmly closed and cut between (see Fig. 4.5).

Top tip

Ensure when cutting the cord, baby's fingers and genitals are clear of the scissors.

Ensure that you are cutting between the two clamps (**see Figure 4.5**).

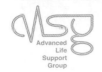

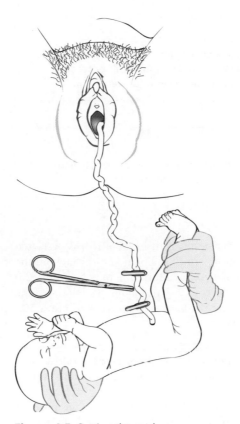

Figure 4.5 Cutting the cord.

If the cord snaps immediately hold and clamp both ends.

Rarely the cord is extremely tight around the neck and the baby cannot deliver through the cord. In this case carefully clamp and divide the cord before delivery of the body. More usually the body can be delivered through the cord.

Delivery of the placenta

- With delivery of the shoulders, give an oxytocic agent (either syntocinon 5 IU IV or, syntocinon 10 IU IM, or IV/IM syntometrine (1 ml vial), or 250 micrograms IV/IM ergometrine or misoprostil 800 micrograms PR).
- Await spontaneous separation of the placenta.
- Signs of separation are:
  ○ cord lengthens
  ○ uterus rises up – on abdominal palpation it is easier to feel
  ○ often a small gush of blood

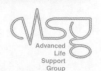

> **Top tips**
>
> Pulling on the cord in an uncontrolled manner may snap the cord or cause a uterine inversion. Therefore, this procedure should only be performed by midwives or obstetricians.

> **Top tips**
>
> In the case of twins or higher multiples ensure all babies are delivered before giving an oxytocic agent.

Pain relief

Entonox is an excellent analgesic agent in labour. It is best used starting from the commencement of the pain and throughout the pain. Deep breaths should be used. "Morphine may be required if the woman is extremely distressed with labour pains (10–20 mg IM). However, be aware that the baby may show signs of respiratory depression at delivery".

Emergency care of delivery in the absence of a midwife

- Help the woman into a comfortable position – all fours, squatting, lying back.
- Do not lie the mother completely flat on her back – propped up is a much better position, or on one side.
- Make a quick assessment of key events (timing should be noted using the 24-hour clock):
  - signs of crowning
  - bleeding
  - ruptured membranes
  - number of weeks
  - number of babies
- The baby should be allowed to deliver spontaneously. However, if there is delay in delivery of the head, the protocol for shoulder dystocia should be immediately instigated (see Chapter 7).
- Document time of delivery of both the head and the body.
- Gently dry and wrap the baby and handover to the mother (Ensure you wrap the baby in a dry towel).
- Keep the baby warm, cover the head – skin-to-skin contact is an excellent method to achieve this.
- If the baby does not breathe spontaneously or remains blue or white, instigate the neonatal resuscitation procedure. (see Chapter 9).

- Obtain midwifery assistance. Ambulance services are required to have policies and procedures in place to obtain midwifery assistance in an emergency. Ensure that you are familiar with these before you need them.

Respiratory rate, pulse and initial blood pressure checks should be performed but in the absence of bleeding or signs of hypertension or shock no further monitoring is required for the first hour, by which time transfer will usually have been achieved.

SUMMARY OF KEY POINTS

- At 8 cm, women are often very distressed and regularly request an epidural or demand that the baby is delivered – this is often one of the most vocal stages.
- Labour is often faster in second and subsequent pregnancies.
- Always consider whether fluid loss could be urine rather than liquor.
- Occasionally membranes will be visible at the vaginal entrance but the presenting part will be much higher and the cervix may not be fully dilated.
- Most babies if left to their own devices will deliver spontaneously without any assistance.
- Pulling too hard on the baby at delivery can cause a brachial plexus injury.
- Ensure when cutting the cord, baby's fingers and genitals are clear of the scissors.
- Ensure that you are cutting between the two clamps and that one clamp really is proximal to the baby and the other is more proximal to the placenta.
- Pulling on the cord in an uncontrolled manner may snap the cord or cause a uterine inversion. Therefore, this procedure should only be performed by midwives or obstetricians.
- In the case of suspected or known twins or higher multiples ensure all babies are delivered before giving oxytocic agent. The presence of twins should be anticipated in the absence of an ultrasound scan if the fundal height is greater than expected following delivery.

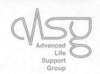
Advanced
Life
Support
Group

CHAPTER 5
Structured approach to the obstetric patient

OBJECTIVES

Having read this chapter, the practitioner should be able to:
• take an obstetric history
• identify the key features of an obstetric history
• perform obstetric primary and secondary surveys

PRIMARY OBSTETRIC SURVEY

Global overview

The obstetric primary survey consists of the first 'hands-on' examination of the pregnant patient. However, the pre-hospital practitioners should, even before beginning the primary survey, have undertaken (almost unconsciously) an initial global overview as they approach the patient. During the global overview, as they walk towards the patient, the practitioner should consider the following:

• Circulation/massive external haemorrhage – This is defined as massive haemorrhage, that is readily visible without the need to disturb the patient's clothing.
• Airway – Is the patient talking (= airway open), or making snoring or gurgling sounds (= airway obstruction), or not making any sounds at all (= altered conscious level or complete airway obstruction)?
• Breathing – Is the patient speaking in whole sentences (no = respiratory or circulatory problem)? What colour is the patient (cyanosis = severe hypoxia)?
• Circulation – What colour is the patient (pale = circulatory problem or pain)?

Pre-Hospital Obstetric Emergency Training, 1st edition. By Malcolm Woollard, Kim Hinshaw, Helen Simpson and Sue Wieteska. Published 2010 by Blackwell Publishing, ISBN: 978-1-4051-8475-5.

- Disability – Is the patient talking, moving, or making sounds (conscious level)?
- Environment – Is there blood on the floor or clothing of the patient? Has the baby been born yet? What position is the patient in? Is the home clean? Is it warm? Are there other children present? Is there clean warm water available?
- Fundus – Does the patient look as if she is in the first, second, or third trimester?
- Get to the point quickly – Start the primary survey.

Primary survey

The obstetric primary survey consists of the first 'hands-on' examination of the pregnant patient. However, it is important to remember there are two patients: neither the mother nor a newly born baby should be overlooked whilst assessing and caring for the other. Both may be at risk, or one may need more urgent attention than the other – it is unlikely to be possible to determine which until a primary survey has been completed on both patients. For the primary survey of newborn babies, see Chapter 9.

The aim of the primary survey is to identify the existence of life-threatening problems, to enable management to be commenced as rapidly as is possible and to reach an early determination of the priority for transportation. The primary survey should be modified in the presence of actual or suspected trauma – see Chapter 10 for specific details.

Circulation/massive external haemorrhage

- Is there a significant volume of blood visible without the need to disturb the patient's clothing?
  - On the floor.
  - Is the patient's clothing soaked?
  - Are there a number of blood-soaked pads in evidence?

Top tip

Massive external haemorrhage, although rare, MUST be managed immediately (if compressible) or the patient may exsanguinate before the primary survey is completed. Spilt blood cannot be replaced in the pre-hospital setting.

Airway

- Is the patient able to talk? (yes = airway open)

- Is the patient making unusual sounds? (gurgling = fluid in the airway requiring suction; snoring = tongue/swelling/foreign body obstruction)
- If the patient is unresponsive, open the airway and look in – suction for fluids, manually remove solid obstructions.

Top tip

If you identify an airway problem, manage this definitively before moving on to the next stage of the primary survey.

If you are unable to open an obstructed airway, get additional advanced airway skills with the shortest possible delay: this is likely to require rapid transportation to the nearest hospital (regardless of the availability of obstetric skills) but *occasionally* you may be able to get help to the scene more quickly for example, BASICS responder with anaesthetic training.

Breathing
- document respiratory rate and effort (Are accessory muscles being used?)
- obtain oxygen saturations as soon as possible
- auscultate for added sounds (wheeze = bronchospasm; coarse sounds = pulmonary oedema)
- assess for the presence of cyanosis
- give oxygen based on clinical findings (not routinely)

Top tip

Increased respiratory rates without increased work of breathing may indicate an attempt to compensate for a circulatory problem.

Top tip

Do NOT give oxygen to 'well' obstetric patients in normal labour. This is not helpful and may alarm the patient unnecessarily.

Top tip

Rates less than 10 or greater than 29 require ventilatory support as they indicate inadequate minute volumes and respiratory failure.

Circulation

- Document radial pulse rate and volume (capillary refill time [CRT] may be used if neither the radial nor carotid pulses can be palpated).
- Assess skin colour and temperature (to touch) (pallor, or cold or damp skin = an adrenergic reaction to shock).
- Assess for bleeding – check underwear, pads, the surface the patient is sitting on, and briefly examine the introitus (the vaginal opening) with the patient's consent and considering their privacy. Ask the patient about bleeding during this problem – if they have discarded pads, how saturated were they? How many pads have they used in what time period?
  - think 'BLOOD ON THE FLOOR AND FIVE MORE':
    - BLOOD ON THE FLOOR – check for visible blood loss again and feel under any clothing or bed linen the patient is sitting or lying on, as this can absorb significant volumes of blood. Look at your gloved hands to see if they are stained with blood.
    - FIVE MORE (look and feel):
      1 Check the introitus for evidence of bleeding (soaked pads or underwear, wounds).
      2 Check the thoracic area for evidence of internal bleeding following trauma (tenderness, wounds, crepitus, patterning from clothes and seatbelts, discolouration).
      3 Check the abdominal area for evidence of internal bleeding (tenderness, guarding, firm woody uterus, wounds, patterning from clothes and seatbelts, discolouration).
      4 Check the pelvis for evidence of injury following trauma (consider mechanism – high speed impact with other significant injuries; complaint of hip or low back pain; bruising. N.B. do not compress or palpate the pelvis as this may dislodge clots).
      5 Check the femurs for signs of fracture following trauma (tenderness, deformity, open fractures).
- Document blood pressure – the systolic is most valuable if you suspect shock.

Top tip

If this is an antepartum haemorrhage (APH) do NOT waste time at this point by inserting cannulae to give fluids: the treatment of APH is surgery in a hospital obstetric unit. Fluids (if indicated) should be started in the ambulance on route to the hospital.

There is NO evidence that pre-hospital IV fluids saves lives: there is good evidence that short on-scene times and pre-alerting the hospital DO save lives.

> **Top tip**
>
> In a full-term patient in labour, any blood loss making a stain larger in diameter than a drinks coaster is cause for significant concern.

Disability

- perform an AVPU assessment of conscious level (Is the patient Alert, responding only to Voice, responding only to Pain, or Unresponsive?)
- document the patient's posture (normal, convulsing [state whether focal or generalised], abnormal flexion, abnormal extension)
- document pupil size and reaction (PEaRL – Pupils Equal and Reacting to Light)

Expose/environment/evaluate

- If you have not already done so, briefly examine the introitus – Is there any evidence of bleeding? Can you see a presenting part of the baby? Is there a prolapsed loop of cord? Have the waters broken? Does the perineum bulge with each contraction? If the baby has been delivered, is there a significant perineal tear? Can you see part of the uterus?
- Is the room warm? Is a newborn at risk of hypothermia? Are the surroundings as clean as you can make them if you are going to deliver on site? Are there other children present (indicates previous pregnancy with live birth)?
- Make an early evaluation about how time critical the patient's problem is. Remember to communicate this clearly to the team, and make sure they have understood and agree with you. If the patient is time critical, decide immediately whether you need to transport the patient urgently to hospital, or whether it is more prudent to treat them at the scene – remember to call for skilled obstetric help if this is the case.

> **Top tip**
>
> It is extremely poor practice to deliver a baby in the back of an ambulance: these have inadequate space, heating, and lighting, and are very unhygienic.

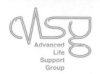

> **Top tip**
>
> Never ignore the concerns of a team member, no matter how junior they are. However senior and experienced you are, you may still miss something important and might even occasionally make mistakes!

Fundus

- Make a quick assessment of fundal height: a fundus at the level of the umbilicus equates to a gestation of approximately 22 weeks. By definition, fundal height below the umbilicus suggests that if the fetus is delivered it is unlikely to survive.

Get to the point quickly

- Remember the aim is to identify time critical problems as quickly as possible, to allow for rapid management and, if appropriate, transportation for definitive care to a suitable obstetric facility. These problems include:
  - significant blood loss at any stage of pregnancy or in the postpartum period
  - cervical shock
  - suspected abruption, placenta praevia, or uterine rupture
  - eclampsia or significant hypertension
  - shoulder dystocia
  - cord prolapse
  - suspected amniotic fluid embolus
  - retained placenta
  - uterine inversion
  - refractory maternal cardiac arrest
  - refractory neonatal cardiac arrest
  - newborn with poor vital signs

  Patients who have one or more of these problems are 'G factor positive'. If transport to hospital is possible, the care provided on scene should be restricted to that necessary to secure the patient's airway, ensure adequate ventilation, and to control significant compressible haemorrhage.

OBSTETRIC SECONDARY SURVEY

If any 'G' factors were identified during the primary survey the secondary survey should only be undertaken when any ABCDE problems have been addressed and transportation to definitive care has commenced (if this is possible). In many cases where the patient is 'G factor positive' it will not be possible or

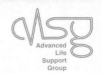

appropriate to undertake a secondary survey in the pre-hospital phase of care.

TAKING AND EVALUATING AN OBSTETRIC HISTORY

Read the patient hand-held maternity notes whenever possible, as this may alert you to any potential obstetric and medical complications which may arise.

Ask the woman or her partner or relative for any information which may be relevant.

Determine:

- The patient's name.
- Date of birth or age.
- The hospital registration number.
- Which hospital the woman has booked for her care in pregnancy, and indeed IF she has booked. Remember it may be a concealed or phantom pregnancy
- Does she have a named obstetric consultant or midwife (the latter will indicate that the mother is booked for low-risk antenatal care)?
- The gestation of pregnancy through the estimated date of delivery (EDD). This may not be possible to determine if the woman has not received any antenatal care or has not booked. You may have to use the last menstrual period (LMP) (if known) as a marker.

If the woman has hand-held notes they may provide a basic history of previous pregnancies and the current pregnancy.

Previous medical history

- Is there a history of hypertension, epilepsy, diabetes, asthma or other major medical or surgical problems that may well have a bearing on the current problem?
- Any history or current use of illicit drugs (this is a leading cause of maternal death).

Past obstetric history

- How many previous pregnancies?
- How many previous deliveries?
- How did she deliver in the past, for example normal delivery or Caesarean section?
- Were there any complications such as bleeding or very early deliveries?

History of current pregnancy

- LMP or gestation
- any problems so far
- number of babies, for example singleton, twins, higher multiple
- care booked with midwife, shared care or consultant-led care
- any concerns with the baby

Top tip

The date of LMP gives a guide to gestation of the pregnancy. In assisted conception this date is likely to be reliable, in natural conception there is a wider scope for error.

History of current problem

Questions should be aimed at clarifying the current problem. Some examples of the types of questions that can be asked are given below (think Labour Pains Discharge Bleeding Fetal Fits):

Labour

- Number of contractions in 10-minute period.
- How strong, how long do they last (seconds/minutes)?
- Feels like pushing.
- Anything hanging between legs – for example a cord.

Pain

- Type – constant, contractions – Does the uterus go hard, coming and going, stabbing, ache?
- Severity – worst pain ever, scale of 0–10.
- Location:
  - abdomen – over uterus, low down, under ribs, one side, back
  - chest – central, one side, back
  - head – frontal, crushing
- Radiation – Does the pain go anywhere else or does it stay in one place?
- Relieving and exacerbating factor – what, if anything, makes the pain worse or better?

Discharge

- colour – clear and odourless, clear and smells of urine, green, yellow, pink, red
- smell
- consistency – watery, thick, jelly-like, frothy
- quantity – gush, trickle, still draining

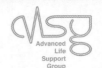

Advanced
Life
Support
Group

Bleeding
- When did it start?
- Quantity: only on wiping after going to toilet, teaspoon, eggcup, soak pants/trousers, sanitary towel, bath towel, blood easily seen running down legs to toes.
- Still bleeding?
- Clots: Are there any and if so how big?
- Is the blood mixed with mucous?

Fetal movements
- Is the baby moving normally?
- Moving less?
- When was the last time she felt the baby move?

Fit
- previous history of fits/epilepsy
- any witnesses
- tonic–clonic movements – How long for?
- associated incontinence, biting tongue/lips
- postictal state

Evaluating the history
- assess history for risk factors
- assess symptom severity
- attempt to make a diagnosis
- use examination findings to confirm diagnosis

See individual chapters for hints regarding risk factors and the significance of signs.

Below are some general hints and clues (Box 5.1)

Box 5.1: Key findings from history and examination

- Severe pain with no fetal movement with or without bleeding – placental abruption until proven otherwise.
- Bleeding that reaches the toes is significant.
- Any bleeding with a low-lying placenta is significant.
- Labour is established if three or more contractions in 10 minutes.
- Rectal pressure may mean she is fully dilated or that the baby is coming down in the OP (occiput posterior position).
- Previous Caesarean section increases the risk of uterine rupture.
- Hypertension increases the risk of abruption.
- If contractions of more than five in 10 minutes consider the diagnosis of abruption.

> ### Box 5.1: Key findings from history and examination (continued)
>
> - Breech presentation and transverse lie have a higher chance of cord prolapse.
> - Previous preterm delivery increases likelihood of another preterm delivery.
> - Twin pregnancies have an increased risk of all obstetric complications.
> - History of a fit in the absence of a history of epilepsy – the woman should be considered to have had an eclamptic fit until proven otherwise (N.B. blood pressure may not be elevated at the time of the fit).
> - Dead babies can 'move' like any immobile object in a pool of fluid (an external movement can cause the baby to knock against the uterine wall and this can be interpreted as a movement).

> ### Top tip
>
> Do not confuse gravidity with parity
> - Gravidity = total number of pregnancies, including current one.
> - Parity = the total number of birth events resulting in a live birth (at any gestation) or a stillbirth (stillbirth is defined as a baby born dead after gestation of more than 24 weeks). A twin delivery is recorded as a single birth event for parity.

Secondary survey

Perform an examination:
- Review the airway.
- Review the breathing: respiratory rate and quality.
- Review the circulation: pulse rate and quality.
- Assess again for blood loss:
  - Look to see how much, note any soaked garments or bed linen. (If yes, why are you doing a secondary survey?)
    - Beware for blood loss down to the toes. (If yes, why are you doing a secondary survey?)
    - Ask to see any visible active bleeding PV by vulval inspection.
    - Is it fresh red bleeding or watery?
    - Are there any clots?
  - Check the blood pressure.

- Review disability – assess GCS, pupils, posture and fits.
- Review your evaluation – Is this still a non-time critical patient?
- If time and the patient's condition permit, undertake a basic obstetric examination.
- Perform an abdominal examination if appropriate. Note any:
  - tenderness
  - rigidity
  - uterine contractions
  - fundal height
  - fetal movements
- If the woman is contracting and is in apparent labour, palpate the contractions for strength and frequency.
- A vulval inspection will be necessary if the woman is feeling the urge to push (or if there has been any concern about PV bleeding).
- Look for the visible signs of the second stage of labour such as:
  - anal dilatation
  - presence of the head (or other presenting part) at the introitus
  - look for the signs of a cord prolapse, particularly if the woman has had a sudden spontaneous rupture of her membranes
- If there has been a spontaneous rupture of membranes. Assess the colour of the liquor. Is it:
  - clear
  - blood stained
  - meconium stained
  - turbid or offensive

  If a vulval inspection is necessary, remember the following:
- **ALWAYS** ask for the woman's consent to perform this inspection, and explain why you need to do it. You should document that you have obtained consent in the notes.
- Explain to the partner or relative accompanying the woman.
- Have someone with you, if possible (ideally another health care practitioner).
- Maintain the woman's dignity. Cover her up immediately following the examination.
- Acknowledge cultural variations, as this forms part of the consent process.
- Respect the woman's right to refuse.

Guidance on the use of internal vaginal examinations

Routine internal vaginal examination by non-obstetric practitioners is never appropriate. It should only be undertaken in extreme obstetric emergencies such as delivery of the after – coming head in a breech presentation, or prolapsed cord.

Measuring blood pressure

This should be performed with the woman in a sitting position, if circumstances allow. The best way of checking a pregnant woman's blood pressure is by using a manual aneroid sphygmomanometer, as this is far more accurate than using an automated device.

This was identified within the CEMACH (2004) report where it was acknowledged that automated blood pressure readings seriously underestimated blood pressure in pre-eclampsia to a significant degree (CEMACH 2004). The diastolic pressure should be documented at the point the sounds disappear (Korotkoff V). Occasionally in pregnancy, the sounds may not disappear. In that circumstance, diastolic BP can be estimated by noting when the sounds become muffled (Korotkoff IV).

A systolic blood pressure of 100 mm Hg is not uncommon in healthy pregnant women. However, as a guide, a systolic blood pressure of less than 90 mm Hg should be acknowledged as indicative of shock if other signs are present. At the other end of the scale, a systolic of 160 mm Hg or over requires urgent medical assessment and treatment, as recommended within the CEMACH (2007c) report.

Always read the patient hand-held records to assess the trend in the woman's blood pressure, and assess for other clinical signs and symptoms for underlying disease or illness.

Fetal assessment

This is limited in the pre-hospital setting, particularly in emergency situations.

Although fetal heart sounds can be heard with a standard stethoscope, they may be difficult to hear, and are not an assurance of fetal well-being. In the cases of placental abruption, fetal heart sounds may be muffled or difficult to hear if there is concealed bleeding within the uterus. Transfer should not be delayed by attempting to auscultate the fetal heart.

Asking the mother about fetal movements is one way of attempting to determine fetal well-being. However, the absence of movements does not indicate a poor outcome. The fetus does not move all of the time and may be in a sleep cycle. The mother may not always feel fetal movements if she is contracting frequently.

Assessing the colour of the liquor if the membranes have ruptured is another way of attempting to assess fetal well-being. If fresh meconium is present in the liquor it will be a yellowy-green colour with particulate matter present. The presence of fresh meconium or heavy blood staining gives cause for concern and alerts the need for appropriate fetal monitoring when the woman is transferred into the hospital setting.

> **Top tip**
>
> Do not delay the transportation of the mother by attempting to determine fetal well-being.

HANDOVER OF THE OBSTETRIC PATIENT

As with all patients handover to another health care practitioner is a crucial point in the management of the patient. If this is not performed correctly important information may be missed, resulting in incorrect or delayed diagnoses and treatment.

A verbal handover should be structured to avoid missing any vital information. Remember that the first stage of the handover process to a hospital may be the pre-alert message and this can use the same structure. ASHICE is one example in current pre-hospital practice and this has been modified to meet the needs of obstetric patients as ASHHIE.

- Age
- Signs and symptoms
  - Be brief, but structure this in the order airway, breathing (include respiratory rate), circulation (bleeding, pulse, BP), disability (AVPU or GCS, pupils, posture, fits), examination (i.e. other pertinent findings, including onset of labour, strength, regularity, duration and intervals between contractions, SROM, show), G factors. Omit any category for which there is no abnormal finding.
- History of the current problem
- History of the current pregnancy
  - gravidity, parity, EDD, and any problems (even if these are not the cause of the current problem)
- Interventions
  - brief description of treatment provided, including timing and doses of any drugs and locations of IV and IO cannulae
- Estimated time of arrival – for pre-alert message

Following verbal handover of the patient all findings and treatment provided must be documented in writing or in electronic format and a copy provided for the attention of obstetric staff and for filing in the patient's hospital notes. If the patient is not hospitalised, the hand-held record should be updated by pre-hospital staff and a copy of their written or printed notes included.

SUMMARY OF KEY POINTS

- Scoop and run is often the way forward with obstetric emergencies.
- If delivery is imminent divert to the nearest unit.
- The obstetric primary survey should be preceded by a global overview.
- The obstetric primary survey aims to identify time critical problems as rapidly as possible. It is similar to any primary survey but includes an assessment of fundal height and places emphasis on the identification of urgent obstetric problems (remember ABCDEFG).
- When examining for haemorrhage, think 'BLOOD ON THE FLOOR AND FIVE MORE'.
- If the patient is 'G Factor Positive' and transportation to hospital is possible, appropriate treatment on scene should be restricted to securing the airway, maintaining adequate ventilation and control of significant haemorrhage.
- Severe pain with no fetal movement with or without bleeding – placental abruption until proven otherwise.
- Bleeding that reaches the toes is significant.
- Any bleeding with a low-lying placenta is significant.
- Labour is established if three or more contractions in 10 minutes.
- Rectal pressure may mean pregnant woman is fully dilated or that the baby is coming down in the OP (occiput posterior position).
- Previous Caesarean section increases the risk of uterine rupture.
- Hypertension increases the risk of abruption.
- If contractions of more than five in 10 minutes consider the diagnosis of abruption.
- Breech presentation and transverse lie have a higher chance of cord prolapse.
- Previous preterm delivery increases likelihood of another preterm delivery.
- Twin pregnancies have an increased risk of all obstetric complications.
- History of a fit in the absence of a history of epilepsy – the woman should be considered to have had an eclamptic fit until proven otherwise (N.B. blood pressure may not be elevated at the time of the fit).
- Dead babies can 'move' like any immobile object in a pool of fluid (an external movement can cause the baby to knock

against the uterine wall and this can be interpreted as a movement).
- Do not delay the transportation of the mother by attempting to determine fetal well-being.
- Verbal handover of the obstetric patient should conform to the ASHHIE structure – Age, Signs and symptoms, History of current problem, History of current pregnancy, Interventions, Estimated time of arrival (for pre-alert).

CHAPTER 6

Emergencies in early pregnancy and complications following gynaecological surgery

---

OBJECTIVES

Having read this chapter, the practitioner should be able to define, identify and describe the pre-hospital management of:
- common complications following gynaecological surgery
- miscarriage
- ectopic pregnancy

ASSESSMENT AND MANAGEMENT OF THE POST-GYNAECOLOGICAL SURGERY PATIENT

The complications of gynaecological surgery are the same as for any type of surgery. Take a full history of the type of surgery and assess symptoms. Some common complications are listed below.

Infection

Urinary tract
- This is a very common type of infection.
- Patients present with:
  - urinary frequency and dysuria
  - loin pain (which may signify pyelonephritis)
  - swinging temperature, sweats and fever
  - feeling unwell
  - nausea and vomiting may occur
- Treatment is with oral antibiotics which can allow them to be managed at home. However, if they have a swinging temperature they will require hospital admission for IV antibiotics.
- If symptoms are mild consider assessment by the GP rather than transporting to hospital.

Pre-Hospital Obstetric Emergency Training, 1st edition. By Malcolm Woollard, Kim Hinshaw, Helen Simpson and Sue Wieteska. Published 2010 by Blackwell Publishing, ISBN: 978-1-4051-8475-5.

Wound infection
- The wound becomes red, hot and inflamed.
- There may be a hardened area above or below the wound where a haematoma has formed.
- The wound may open slightly allowing pus to drain out.
- Pain can also be experienced at the wound site.
- A temperature will be present (this may be swinging) and the woman may feel generally unwell.
- Rarely the whole wound and the sheath itself will open producing a burst abdomen. Bowel may be seen through the opening:
  - cover the wound with a moist clean occlusive dressing and transport to hospital immediately
- Most other wounds should have a dry dressing applied. Consider assessment and treatment in the pre-hospital setting rather than transporting to hospital.
- Gas gangrene should be suspected if the wound looks necrotic or there are blisters on the skin surface. Transport to hospital for assessment.
- Treatment is with antibiotics usually given orally. Immediate repair of the wound is usually not advisable as it will break down again.

Bleeding
- following hysterectomy if a vault haematoma develops or a pedicle slips there may be significant haemorrhage from the vagina
- assess severity according to haemorrhage criteria

Pulmonary embolism
- take a full history of the type of surgery and assess symptoms
- there may be a history of calf pain or sudden collapse
- risk factors include extensive pelvic surgery, obesity, smoking, previous PE
- assess ABC, maintain airway and consider intubation if required
- instigate CPR if no cardiac output
- immediate transfer to nearest emergency department
- IV access with two large-bore cannulae on route to hospital
- consider thrombolysis (if available)

Bowel perforation and paralytic ileus
- both may occur after surgery often 2–5 days following the procedure
- paralytic ileus is more common
- bowel perforation should be suspected after any laparoscopic procedure
- there is a history of nausea and vomiting, abdominal distension, not passing wind or defaecating

- bowel sounds may be absent on auscultation of the abdomen, and may also be tympanic on percussion
- with bowel perforation, signs of overt peritonitis may be apparent (right abdomen)
- assess ABC, provide analgesia, transport to the nearest emergency department, IV access on route

MISCARRIAGE

Definition

Miscarriage is the loss of a pregnancy before 24 completed weeks. It can occur in either the first or second trimester, the further advanced the pregnancy the more bleeding can occur. Miscarriage is more common in the first 12 weeks.

There are different types of miscarriage:
- Incomplete: the cervix will be open and some of fetal/placental tissue passed but some will still be in the uterine cavity. Bleeding can be heavy or light.
- Inevitable: cervix open but no tissue passed at present. Bleeding can be heavy or light.
- Complete: all the placental/fetal tissue has passed and the cervix will be closed or closing and bleeding will be settling.
- Threatened: there has been some bleeding but no tissue has been passed and on ultrasound assessment the fetus is thought to still be viable.
- Missed: there has been very little or no bleeding and on ultrasound assessment the fetus is either dead or has not developed properly.
- Septic miscarriage: this occurs when infection follows any miscarriage. It can be associated with incomplete miscarriage, post-surgical evacuation or following termination of pregnancy. Signs and symptoms include:
  - bleeding and abdominal pain
  - shock (usually septic shock)
  - headache
  - nausea
  - hot and cold flushes
  - sweating
  - shivering
  - rise in pulse and temperature
  - vaginal loss can be offensive

To make an accurate diagnosis of the type of miscarriage, vaginal examination and ultrasound are required: neither is appropriate in the pre-hospital setting. In the acute situation, management depends on the clinical situation rather than the absolute diagnosis.

CERVICAL SHOCK

This occurs when some products of conception are partly passed through the cervix and become 'trapped'. The level of shock is often out of proportion to the amount of blood loss.

Top tip

Cervical shock is a life-threatening emergency which requires urgent obstetric intervention to resolve. These patients should be transported to hospital without delay (lights and sirens) with IV fluids given on route.

Risk factors
- previous history of miscarriage
- previously identified potential miscarriage at scan
- smoker
- obesity

Diagnosis

Clinical history
- bleeding can be light or very heavy
- there may be a history of passing clots or jelly-like tissue. Any tissue that has been passed and collected should be brought to hospital
- pain – central, period-like cramps can radiate to back or down legs
- symptoms of pregnancy may be subsiding such as nausea or breast tenderness
- not associated with shoulder tip pain or diarrhoea (this would indicate potential ectopic pregnancy)
- if bleeding and pain are improving more likely to be complete or threatened miscarriage

---

Top tip

Any tissue that has been passed and collected should be brought to hospital.

Pre-hospital management
- open, maintain and protect the airway in accordance with the patient's clinical need
- If oxygen saturation on air falls below 94% give oxygen. If SpO_2 is less than 85% use non-rebreathing mask; otherwise use a simple face mask. Aim for a target saturation of 94–98%.

- assess and document:
  - ○ respiratory rate
  - ○ pulse rate and quality
  - ○ CRT or blood pressure
  - ○ obstetric history
- to assess quantity of blood loss:
  - ○ blood at the toes
  - ○ blood loss on pad
  - ○ blood on clothes
  - ○ blood on bed sheets
- initiate transfer to hospital and inform of arrival
- site one or two large-bore (14 G) IV cannulae on route to hospital
- commence IV fluid (250 ml aliquots) to maintain a systolic BP of 100 mm Hg
- administer analgesia as appropriate
- maintain nil by mouth
- bradycardia secondary to cervical shock can be treated with atropine (500 microgram repeated up to 3 mg)

Suggestion

If there is light bleeding or bleeding that has resolved, with no associated pain – contact hospital and consider booking for an evaluation in either an outpatient or early pregnancy assessment unit.

Top tip

If shock is out of proportion to bleeding consider ectopic or cervical shock.

Top tip

Periods can be late on occasion. To determine pregnancy ask:
- Is the bleeding like a normal period?
- Is the LMP <6 weeks ago?
- Has there been a positive pregnancy test?

Top tip

Ectopic bleeding tends to be:
- lighter
- pain tends to be more to one side
- may be associated with shoulder tip pain or diarrhoea

> **Top tip**
>
> - In the event of life-threatening bleeding with evidence that products of conception have definitely been passed a dose of ergometrine 500 microgram IV can be given.
> - Alternatively, misoprostol 800 microgram PR can be given.
> - Liaise with the on call gynaecologist as a second dose of either may occasionally be required.

ECTOPIC PREGNANCY

Definition

An ectopic pregnancy is a pregnancy that has implanted somewhere other than in the uterine cavity – normally in the fallopian tube but can rarely implant on the ovary or elsewhere in the abdominal cavity (Fig. 6.1). Ectopic pregnancy is increasing in frequency, and complicates between 1–2% of all pregnancies.

Risk factors
- pelvic inflammatory disease
- intrauterine contraceptive device
- infertility
- previous ectopic
- tubal surgery
- sterilisation
- reversal of sterilisation
- endometriosis

Diagnosis

Clinical history
- shoulder tip pain
- usually 6–8 weeks pregnant

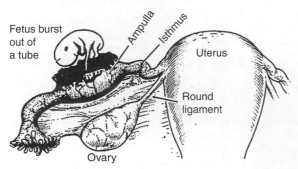

Figure 6.1 Diagram of uterus/tubes/ovaries and possible sites of implantation.

- diarrhoea
- pain on defecation/rectal pain
- postural hypotension
- shock
- vaginal bleeding/spotting
- history of dizziness
- fainting
- tachycardia

Examination findings
- tenderness on one side
- rebound
- adnexal tenderness
- shock
- bleeding (this may be absent)
- light or heavy menstrual bleeding

Biochemical markers
There will be women being monitored in the community with serial βhCG measurements who are considered to be at risk of ectopic pregnancy. Check with the patient to determine if this is the case.

Top tip

No single component is likely to diagnose an ectopic pregnancy in isolation – the complete picture is more important. Thus in the acute pre-hospital situation a clinical suspicion of an ectopic is all that is possible.

Top tip

Asymptomatic women can have ectopic pregnancies; however, these would not present in the acute situation (ultrasound diagnosis is required).
The fact that a period has not been missed does not exclude an ectopic but on closer questioning the last period was often lighter than normal.
Ectopic pregnancy can present with atypical urinary or bowel symptoms (eg diarrhoea, pain on defecation) Maternal deaths from ruptured ectopic have occurred when these symptoms were ignored.

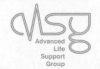

Top tip

Shock can develop and is often severe and out of proportion to the amount of vaginal blood loss.
Cardiovascular instability should be taken seriously.
Women who die of ectopic pregnancy die from blood loss.
Urgent action is therefore indicated in such cases.

Pre-hospital management

- open, maintain and protect the airway in accordance with the patient's clinical need
- If oxygen saturation on air falls below 94% give oxygen. If SpO_2 is less than 85% use non-rebreathing mask; otherwise use a simple face mask. Aim for a target saturation of 94–98%.
- assess and document:
  - respiratory rate
  - pulse rate and quality
  - CRT or blood pressure
  - obstetric history
- transport without delay to appropriate hospital facility for example ED/early pregnancy assessment unit as agreed
- site one or two large-bore (14 G) IV cannulae on route to hospital
- commence IV fluid (250 ml aliquots) to maintain a systolic BP of 100 mm Hg
- administer analgesia as appropriate
- maintain nil by mouth

Top tip

If already shocked, this is a life-threatening situation and speed is of the essence, a full history from a family member on route is always useful in these situations.

Top tip

Remember shoulder tip pain, diarrhoea and pain on defaecation.

Advanced
Life
Support
Group

Top tip

Vaginal bleeding can be absent, light or heavy, although heavier loss is more often associated with miscarriage.

SUMMARY OF KEY POINTS

In miscarriage:
- Cervical shock is a life-threatening emergency which requires urgent obstetric intervention to resolve. These patients should be transported to hospital without delay (lights and sirens) with IV fluids given on route.
- Any tissue that has been passed and collected should be brought to hospital.
- If shock is out of proportion to bleeding consider ectopic or cervical shock.
- In the event of life-threatening bleeding and there is evidence that products of conception have been passed a dose of ergometrine 500 microgram IV can be given.
- Alternatively misoprostol 800 microgram pr can be given.

In ectopic pregnancy:
- No single component is likely to diagnose an ectopic pregnancy in isolation – the complete picture is more important. Thus in the acute pre-hospital situation, a clinical suspicion of an ectopic is all that is possible.
- Asymptomatic women can have ectopic pregnancies; however, these would not present in the acute situation (ultrasound diagnosis is required).
- An absence of amenorrhoea does not exclude an ectopic but on closer questioning the last period was often lighter than normal.
- Ectopic pregnancy can present with atypical urinary or bowel symptoms (eg diarrhoea, pain on defaecation). Maternal deaths from ruptured ectopic have occurred when these symptoms were ignored.
- If already shocked, ectopic pregnancy is a life-threatening situation and speed is of the essence, a full history from a family member on route is always useful in these situations.
- Remember shoulder tip pain, diarrhoea and pain on defaecation can indicate ectopic pregnancy.
- Vaginal bleeding can be absent, light or heavy in ectopic pregnancy, although heavier loss is more often associated with miscarriage.

CHAPTER 7
Emergencies in late pregnancy

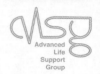

OBJECTIVES

This chapter addresses the recognition and management of emergencies in the later stages of pregnancy, including the first and second stages of labour – up to and including delivery of the baby.

Having read this chapter, the practitioner should be able to define, identify and describe the pre-hospital management of:

- pregnancy-induced hypertension (PIH), pre-eclampsia and eclampsia, haemolysis-elevated liver enzymes and low platelets (HELLP) and acute fatty liver of pregnancy (AFLP)
- preterm labour
- antepartum haemorrhage (APH), including placenta praevia and placental abruption
- uterine rupture
- abnormal presentations and lies
- multiple pregnancy
- shoulder dystocia
- umbilical cord problems, including short and prolapsed cord and cord rupture
- amniotic fluid embolus

HYPERTENSION IN PREGNANCY

Introduction

Hypertension from all causes is the commonest medical problem in pregnancy and affects between 10 and 15% of all pregnancies. It is a heterogeneous group of conditions and includes PIH, pre-existing (for example 'essential') hypertension, pre-eclampsia and eclampsia. The two conditions of HELLP syndrome and AFLP

Pre-Hospital Obstetric Emergency Training, 1st edition. By Malcolm Woollard, Kim Hinshaw, Helen Simpson and Sue Wieteska. Published 2010 by Blackwell Publishing, ISBN: 978-1-4051-8475-5.

are felt to be part of the spectrum of disease that includes pre-eclampsia and eclampsia.

Pre-existing hypertension

Definition

Women may enter pregnancy with pre-existing hypertension due to an underlying cause. If hypertension is detected before 13 weeks, this is likely to reflect pre-existing hypertension. Hypertension in a young person may only be detected for the first time in early pregnancy. At some point, this will require formal investigation to exclude an underlying cause (for example renal or cardiac disease or Cushing's syndrome). However, most will not have a defined cause and fall under the category of mild 'essential' hypertension. These women are at increased risk of developing superimposed pre-eclampsia and fetal growth restriction. The risk is almost 50% if there is severe hypertension in early pregnancy (diastolic BP >110 mm Hg). Again, they require close monitoring in order to detect complications, and in particular the development of pre-eclampsia or growth restriction.

Risk factors

- renal disease
- diabetes
- obesity
- advanced maternal age (over 40 years)
- pre-existing cardiovascular disease
- hypertension on the oral contraceptive pill
- Cushing's disease

Pregnancy-induced hypertension

Definition

PIH is a generic term used to define a significant rise in blood pressure occurring after 20 weeks **in the absence of proteinuria or other features of pre-eclampsia**. It is usually mild with blood pressure levels of around 140/90. About 15% of women who present with PIH will develop pre-eclampsia. Earlier onset of PIH (around 20–24 weeks) results in a 40% risk of developing pre-eclampsia, whereas mild rises in BP beyond 37 weeks are only associated with a 10% risk of developing the disease. Women with uncomplicated PIH require close monitoring in the antenatal period to pick up those who are going to develop pre-eclampsia. If PIH is uncomplicated by pre-eclampsia, the maternal and fetal outcomes are good. PIH may recur in subsequent pregnancies.

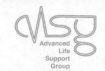

Risk factors
- primiparity or first child with a new partner
- previous severe pre-eclampsia
- essential hypertension
- diabetes
- obesity
- renal disease
- advanced maternal age (over 40 years)
- pre-existing cardiovascular disease
- Cushing's disease

Pre-eclampsia

Definition
Pre-eclampsia is hypertension associated with proteinuria developing after 20 weeks' gestation. It may also be associated with excessive peripheral oedema. It should be noted that some degree of oedema is common in almost all pregnant women. However, oedema of the fingers and face is much more likely to represent pre-eclampsia, than swelling of the lower limbs. It can occur as early as 20 weeks but more commonly occurs beyond 24–28 weeks. It is more common in first pregnancies where 1 in 10 women will develop pre-eclampsia. The incidence of severe pre-eclampsia is approximately 1% of all pregnancies.

The underlying pathophysiology is not fully understood. However, it is known that the placenta plays an important role, such that the normal physiological changes that occur in the vessels of the uterus do not occur. This is thought to be related to either abnormal endothelial function (the lining of small vessels) or a factor produced by trophoblast (placental cells). This leads to poor perfusion of the placenta resulting in a fetus which is growth-restricted.

In the 2007 CEMACH report, pre-eclampsia accounted for 18/132 (13.6%) of maternal deaths related to direct pregnancy causes. It remains the second leading cause of maternal death (equal with sepsis) in the UK (CEMACH 2007c).

Risk factors
- primiparity or first child with a new partner
- previous severe pre-eclampsia
- essential hypertension
- diabetes
- obesity
- twins or higher multiples
- renal disease
- advanced maternal age (over 40 years)

- young maternal age (less than 16 years)
- pre-existing cardiovascular disease
- Cushing's disease

Diagnosis

The disease may be of mild, moderate or severe degree. Women with mild to moderate pre-eclampsia are asymptomatic and the disease is usually diagnosed at routine antenatal visits. This is often managed on an outpatient basis initially, with regular review on the obstetric day unit. However, it may require admission to hospital and early delivery if the disease progresses. In the UK, the diagnosis of pre-eclampsia includes an increase in blood pressure (above 140/90), detection of protein in the patient's urine and sometimes oedema.

When measuring blood pressure, the woman should be semi-recumbent and an appropriately sized cuff should be used. In women with a larger arm, using a normal-sized cuff may result in falsely high BP readings. It is important to record both systolic and diastolic pressures. The latter should be assessed using Korotkoff V (that is sound disappearance). Korotkoff IV (that is 'muffling') should only be used if heart sounds do not disappear as pressure readings fall to zero.

Severe pre-eclampsia may present in a patient with known mild pre-eclampsia or may present with little prior warning. The blood pressure is significantly raised (160/110) with proteinuria and one or more of the following symptoms and signs:

- headache – severe and frontal
- visual disturbances
- epigastric pain (due to stretching of the liver capsule) – often mistaken for heartburn
- right-sided upper abdominal pain – due to stretching of the liver capsule
- muscle twitching or tremor
- other symptoms – nausea, vomiting, confusion
- rapidly progressive oedema
- severe pre-eclampsia is a 'multi-organ' disease – although hypertension is a cardinal feature, other complications include:
  ○ intracranial haemorrhage
  ○ stroke
  ○ renal failure
  ○ liver failure
  ○ abnormal blood clotting such as disseminated intravascular coagulation (DIC)
  ○ placental abruption and associated massive haemorrhage

One of the 'top ten recommendations' in the recent CEMACH report highlighted the importance of aggressive treatment of high systolic blood pressure (SBP 160 mm Hg or more) in order to reduce the chance of maternal intracerebral bleeding and stroke (CEMACH 2007c). Therefore, these mothers require immediate admission to an appropriate obstetric unit.

Pre-hospital management

Pre-hospital care practitioners will not usually be involved with management of mild PIH or mild pre-eclampsia. However, it is important that any pregnant women should have their blood pressure checked during assessment, even if they do not have suspicious symptoms. A new finding of BP 140/90 or higher requires review by a midwife or discussion with the local obstetric unit to decide if admission is necessary. **A new systolic BP of 160 or a diastolic of 110 or higher should trigger automatic admission to an obstetric unit**. A review of their hand-held maternity notes will highlight any changes in BP over the preceding weeks.

The following recommendations relate to management of women with severe pre-eclampsia:

1 review ABCDEFGs
2 review whether there are any 'time-critical' features requiring rapid transfer:
   o headache – severe and frontal
   o visual disturbances
   o epigastric pain
   o right-sided upper abdominal pain
   o muscle twitching or tremor
   o confusion
3 inform hospital of impending arrival
4 secure venous access on route to hospital, in case IV medication is required (see 'eclampsia' below)
5 **DO NOT** give routine IV fluids as these patients are at risk of developing acute pulmonary oedema, even with small boluses of crystalloid. If fluids are attached to the cannula, the flow rate should be no more than 80 ml/h (use normal saline or Hartman's, but not dextrose in water)

Top tip

Restrict IV fluids to a maximum of 80 ml/h to avoid pulmonary oedema.

Avoid ergometrine/syntometrine in the third stage of labour, as it may precipitate severe hypertension and intracerebral bleeding.

> **Top tip**
>
> Syntocinon 10 IU IM or 800 micrograms PR can be given if there is significant third-stage bleeding.

Eclampsia

Definition

Eclampsia is defined as tonic–clonic, generalised 'grand mal' seizures, usually in association with signs or symptoms of pre-eclampsia. It is one of the most dangerous complications of pregnancy with a mortality rate of 2% in the UK. It occurs in about 2.7:10,000 deliveries, usually beyond 24 weeks (UKOSS 2007). Many patients will have had pre-existing pre-eclampsia (of mild, moderate or severe degree), **but cases of eclampsia can present acutely with no prior warning**. One-third of cases present for the first time post-delivery (usually in the first 48 hours).

Although eclampsia is often preceded by severe pre-eclampsia: in many cases the blood pressure will only be mildly elevated at presentation (140/80 to 90).

The hypoxia caused during a grand mal seizure may lead to significant fetal compromise and even death. There is a risk of placental abruption and massive haemorrhage. Occasionally, there may be cortical blindness after an eclamptic fit. Fitting is usually self-limiting, but may be prolonged and repeated.

Other complications associated with eclampsia include renal failure, hepatic failure and DIC.

> **Top tip**
>
> Always assume that a grand mal seizure in pregnancy (beyond 20 weeks) is due to eclampsia until proven otherwise.

Risk factors
- known pre-eclampsia
- primiparity or first child with a new partner
- previous severe pre-eclampsia
- essential hypertension
- diabetes
- obesity
- twins or higher multiples
- renal disease
- advanced maternal age (over 40 years)
- young maternal age (less than 16 years)
- pre-existing cardiovascular disease
- Cushing's disease

Diagnosis

The presence or history of a tonic–clonic fit after 20 weeks of pregnancy.

> **Top tip**
>
> Epileptic patients can have tonic–clonic fits. If after 20 weeks of pregnancy a fitting epileptic patient has a history of hypertension or pre-eclampsia, treat as for eclampsia. If there is no hypertension or pre-eclampsia treat for epilepsy, but monitor blood pressure until after the postictal phase and discuss with midwife.

Pre-hospital management

1 Proceed with the patient in 15–30° left lateral tilt or the left lateral (recovery) position.
2 Open, maintain and protect the airway in accordance with the patient's clinical need.
3 If oxygen saturation on air falls below 94% give oxygen. If SpO_2 is less than 85% use non-rebreathing mask; otherwise use a simple face mask. Aim for a target saturation of 94–98%.
4 If the mother has continuous or recurrent fits, secure venous or IO access (DO NOT give IV fluid boluses because of the risk of provoking pulmonary oedema). Otherwise postpone obtaining access until on route to hospital.
5 This is a 'time-critical' situation and transport to hospital should be arranged at the earliest opportunity.
6 Inform hospital of impending arrival.
7 The definitive treatment of eclampsia, either to treat ongoing or recurrent fits, or to prevent further fits occurring is magnesium sulphate a 4-g loading dose IV or IO over 15 minutes (this would then be followed by an infusion of 1 g/h on arrival at hospital).
8 **If magnesium sulphate is unavailable and the patient is in status** epilepticus, consider diazemuls 10–20 mg IV or IO titrated against effect or rectal diazepam 10–20 mg.

> **Top tip**
>
> Usually eclamptic fits are single and self-limiting lasting for approximately 2 minutes. The definitive treatment is magnesium sulphate to prevent further fits.
>
> If magnesium sulphate is unavailable, avoid using diazepam or other benzodiazepines unless the fits are prolonged or recur (see Fig. 7.1).

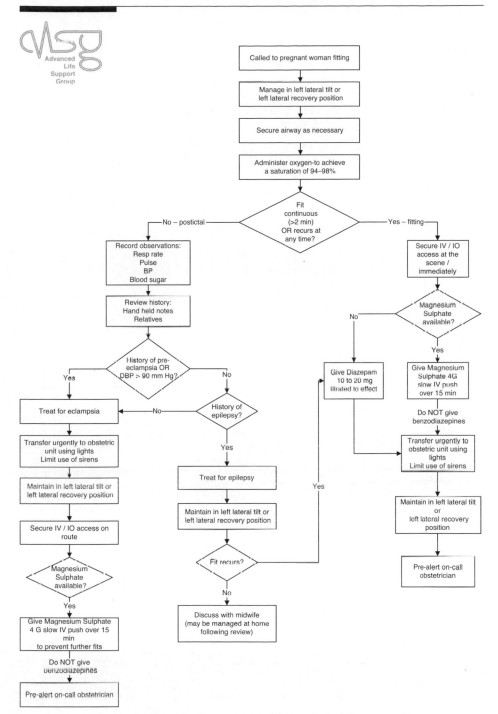

Figure 7.1 Management of fits in pregnancy.

> **Top tip**
>
> The use of sirens may precipitate further convulsions or an increase in the patient's blood pressure; therefore, their use should be avoided if at all possible. Rapid progress to hospital with lights is paramount.

HELLP syndrome

Definition

This is a syndrome related to pre-eclampsia (haemolysis, elevated liver enzymes, low platelets). This is more common in multigravid patients and presents with:

- mild hypertension (140/90)
- right upper quadrant or epigastric pain (65%)
- nausea and vomiting (35%)
- placental abruption (15%)
- liver rupture (rare)

Risk factors

- known pre-eclampsia
- multiparity
- previous history of HELLP

Diagnosis

This will not be diagnosed in the pre-hospital setting; however, you may have a suspicion based on symptoms.

Pre-hospital management

Management in the pre-hospital situation is the same as for severe pre-eclampsia.

Acute fatty liver of pregnancy

Definition

AFLP is a rare condition (1 in 10,000 pregnancies) but has a high maternal mortality (10–20%) and fetal mortality (20–30%). Presentation is usually nearer 37 weeks and the cardinal symptom is severe nausea, vomiting, malaise and mild jaundice. Features of mild pre-eclampsia may be present. Pre-hospital care is the same as for severe pre-eclampsia. Management in hospital is supportive with prompt delivery (induction of labour or Caesarean section).

Risk factors

- first pregnancy
- obesity
- male fetuses

Diagnosis
This will not be diagnosed in the pre-hospital setting; however, you may have a suspicion based on symptoms. A low BM result would raise the index of suspicion.

Pre-hospital management
Management in the pre-hospital situation is the same as for severe pre-eclampsia.

PRETERM LABOUR

Definition
Preterm labour is defined as labour occurring more than 3 weeks before the expected date of delivery – that is, before the completion of 37 weeks of pregnancy. Preterm labour is a significant predictor of neonatal morbidity and mortality, and survival of newborns delivered before the 24th week of pregnancy is unusual, although not impossible. In 2005, 58% of babies born at 24 weeks' gestation survived the first 28 days of life, increasing to 77% at 25 weeks' gestation and 92% at 27–28 weeks' gestation (CEMACH 2007c).

Risk factors
- previous preterm labour
- twins or higher multiples
- smoking
- low socioeconomic groups
- previous suspected cervical incompetence
- known SROM in this pregnancy

Diagnosis
The signs and symptoms may be similar to that of normal labour, although there may be little or no contraction pain and the membranes may rupture before the onset of labour. Malpresentations – such as breech presentation – are common. It is unlikely that the head has engaged before labour starts, and if the membranes have ruptured, the practitioner should be aware of the possibility of cord prolapse.

Top tip

Preterm labour can proceed rapidly to delivery: a careful assessment may prevent the need to deliver in the back of an ambulance.

Abnormal presentations and prolapsed cord are more common than with term labour.

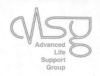

- Assess the patient using the ABCDEFG primary survey.
- Assess the fundal height – remember if the fundus is below the umbilicus this is equivalent to a pregnancy of approximately 24 weeks, and the fetus is unlikely to be viable.
- In particular, remember to get to the point quickly and attempt to identify time-critical problems:
  - abnormal presentation
  - prolapsed cord
  - maternal haemorrhage
- Determine if birth appears to be imminent as this will affect your management plan, and as always obtain an obstetric history from the mother and by reviewing her patient-held records.

Pre-hospital management

1 If your assessment indicates that you can guarantee arriving at the hospital before delivery, commence transportation without delay as a time-critical (lights and sirens) transfer. **Remember to inform the maternity unit of your impending arrival**.

2 DO NOT commence transportation if the birth appears to be imminent or you assess that it will occur before your arrival at hospital:

   2.1 Request the attendance of a midwife at the scene.

   2.2 Request the attendance of a second ambulance to provide additional personal, allowing separate management of mother and baby after delivery and, if necessary, separate transportation. Ideally, this second ambulance should bring an incubator, but obtaining this should not be permitted to significantly delay its arrival at the incident.

   2.3 Remember you will have two patients, so you will need maternity and paediatric (neonatal) kits, oxygen, entonox, ALS kit, and warm towels and blankets. Make sure all appropriate kit is available and laid out – prepare a separate area for management of the baby, avoiding drafts if possible.

   2.4 Manage delivery as you would for term labour (see Chapter 4), but be prepared for abnormal presentations and cord prolapse. The probability of needing to provide ventilatory or circulatory support to the preterm baby is also higher than with a term delivery (see Chapter 9).

   2.5 Maintaining the temperature of the newly born preterm baby is essential: hypothermia can occur rapidly and is associated with significant morbidity. Remember to dry the baby vigorously and wrap them in clean towels and ensure the head is covered. Only the face should remain exposed. Almost all resuscitative measures can and should be performed without the need to expose the newborn.

2.6 Carefully assess the baby in accordance with standard procedures. If resuscitation is necessary, follow the guidelines for newborn life support (see Chapter 9).

Top tip

Request the attendance of a second ambulance *immediately* you decide not to move the mother and at the same time as you request the attendance of a midwife. This will provide additional resources to permit separate care and transportation of mother and baby.

Top tip

Ensure that appropriate measures are taken to ensure the baby is kept warm *immediately* they are born and before resuscitation interventions are undertaken. CPR and ALS will be ineffective if the baby is allowed to become hypothermic, and this is a particular risk in the pre-hospital setting.

Top tip

Ensure that you monitor both mother and baby post-delivery. It is very easy to get distracted by the need to care for a small newborn at the cost of missing a significant post-APH. Similarly, a distressed or ill mother may distract you from caring for the baby for long enough to allow the child to become hypothermic.

ANTEPARTUM HAEMORRHAGE

Definition

APH is defined as bleeding from the vagina before labour but after 24 completed weeks of pregnancy. The volume of blood lost can be just a few millilitres, and in most cases this is not indicative of a serious problem. However, it is vital that even if blood loss is minimal, the patient is assessed and monitored carefully as, occasionally, a small amount of external blood loss may be associated with significant internal (concealed) haemorrhage as in the case of a placental abruption (see later).

Significant external haemorrhage of 1 L or more can also occur, and this is commonly associated with placenta praevia (see later). Massive APH is the cause of 8.4% of stillbirths in the UK

(CEMACH 2007b). Maternal death from APH is rare – in the period 2000–2002, there were only seven cases (CEMACH 2004). However, APH can weaken the mother's ability to cope with a postpartum haemorrhage (PPH).

Top tip

A small amount of blood lost externally may indicate a massive concealed haemorrhage: any volume of external blood loss greater than that of a show (blood loss more than the size of a coaster) should alert the practitioner to the risk of serious hidden bleeding.

Risk factors
- maternal age over 40 years
- the presence of complex medical disorders before pregnancy
- multigravida
- previous Caesarean section resulting in placenta praevia or accreta (abnormal adherence of part or all of the placenta to the uterine wall)
- known placenta praevia
- previous history of abruption
- use of crack cocaine can precipitate abruption
- coagulopathies

Diagnosis
External blood loss that even slightly exceeds the quantity of a normal 'show' should be treated with suspicion. A thorough ABCDEFG approach should be applied to patient assessment and ongoing monitoring. The practitioner should anticipate the possibility of a minor bleed being associated with ongoing concealed bleeding or a subsequent catastrophic revealed haemorrhage. If the vital signs indicate shock then this should precipitate appropriate management regardless of the quantity of blood that has been seen; however, up to 50% of the maternal blood volume can be lost without a concomitant fall in blood pressure or increase in heart rate.

Top tip

Pregnant patients may lose up to 50% of their blood volume without a change in their blood pressure or heart rate.

Pre-hospital management
This is a time-critical life-threatening emergency requiring rapid lights and sirens transport to hospital.

The generic treatment for an APH is the same regardless of whether it is concealed or revealed.

Whilst performing an obstetric primary survey and obtaining an obstetric history:

1 open, maintain and protect the airway in accordance with the patient's clinical need
2 If oxygen saturation on air falls below 94% give oxygen. If SpO_2 is less than 85% use non-rebreathing mask; otherwise use a simple face mask. Aim for a target saturation of 94–98%.
3 remember to position the mother in the 15–30° left lateral position to avoid further compromise of the fetal circulation due to vena caval compression by the uterus
4 start transportation without delay to a hospital with staffed obstetric theatres, blood transfusion, ICU and anaesthetic services immediately available
5 inform the senior on-call obstetrician of your impending arrival
6 insert one or two large-bore (14 G) cannulae on route (do NOT delay on scene to do this). If it is not possible to gain IV access, consider using an intraosseous cannula
7 administer crystalloids in 250 ml aliquots to maintain an SBP of 100 mm Hg. Do NOT administer further 250 ml aliquots once the SBP reaches 100 mm Hg as this may increase the risk of re-bleeding due to clot disruption. Watch closely for further signs of circulatory decompensation
8 administer analgesia if the patient is in pain – use morphine cautiously if the patient is hypotensive
9 give nothing by mouth as the patient may require anaesthesia and surgery

---

Top tip

Do NOT waste time on scene to start IVs: **the treatment of massive APH is surgery**.

Top tip

Hypotensive resuscitation is NOT appropriate in managing hypovolaemic shock in pregnant patients.

Top tip

The three interventions most likely to save the lives of mother and baby are:
1 rapid (lights and sirens) transportation

2 selecting a receiving hospital with staffed obstetric theatres, blood transfusion, ICU and anaesthetic services immediately available

3 pre-alerting the senior on-call obstetrician

Top tip

Have a high index of suspicion of concealed haemorrhage in the presence of an appropriate history and altered mental status or dysrhythmias (particularly worsening tachycardia) regardless of the SBP.

Top tip

In the event of external haemorrhage exceeding 500 ml, be prepared to give IV fluids as SBP may fall precipitously at any time.

Top tip

In the urgency of managing a serious haemorrhage **do not forget to position the mother to avoid vena caval compression by the uterus.**

PLACENTAL ABRUPTION

Definition
Placental abruption is defined as separation of a normally sited placenta from the uterine wall, resulting in bleeding from the maternal sinuses. Haemorrhage is commonly entirely or partially concealed, as blood can only escape through the genital canal if it tracks down behind the membranes. The muscle wall of the uterus itself can also be infiltrated with blood (Couvelaire). However, total blood loss is likely to be significant. The severity of shock can be sufficiently severe to result in maternal coagulopathies (for example DIC) and renal failure. Two women died of abruption between 2003 and 2005 (CEMACH 2007c).

Risk factors
- maternal age over 40 years
- the presence of complex medical disorders before pregnancy

- multigravida
- previous history of abruption
- use of crack cocaine can precipitate abruption
- coagulopathies
- PIH/essential hypertension
- road traffic collisions/significant abdominal trauma

Diagnosis

Conduct a thorough ABCDEFG primary survey and obtain an obstetric history: abruption can be associated with severe PIH. Note that placental abruption can occur at any point in a pregnancy. In contrast to placenta praevia, an abruption commonly results in very severe abdominal pain. The patient may describe this as a contraction that never goes away. If the patient is not already in labour, contractions are likely to start, but this will be difficult to assess as the uterus is tense and abdominal tenderness will be present. On palpation the uterus will feel hard and woody.

The volume of blood lost is likely to be dramatically underestimated: any revealed bleeding may be dark in colour as it may have de-saturated during its slowed passage to the cervical canal. The volume of blood lost and the loss of the maternal–fetal circulation arising from significant separation of the placenta can result in intrauterine death (see Fig. 7.2).

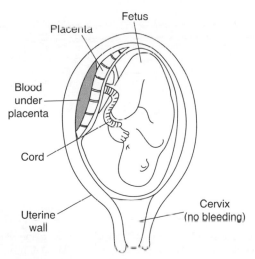

Figure 7.2 Concealed abruption: here all of the bleeding is under the placenta, pain is significant and uterus tender, no revealed bleeding.

> **Top tip**
>
> Do not underestimate the severity of the problem by relying on revealed blood loss alone. If the patient appears to be shocked with minimal external haemorrhage and a painful tense uterus, always assume placental abruption.

Pre-hospital management

If you suspect placental abruption, **this is a time-critical emergency: rapid (lights and sirens) transportation to hospital is vital**. Both mother and fetus are at risk, although the baby is likely to die before the mother. Tactfully ask the mother when she last felt the baby move and remember to pass this information to the receiving obstetrician. Follow the generic treatment guidelines for APH (see page 75).

PLACENTA PRAEVIA

Definition

Placenta praevia is defined as a placenta completely or partially situated in the lower part of the uterus. Separation of the placenta can

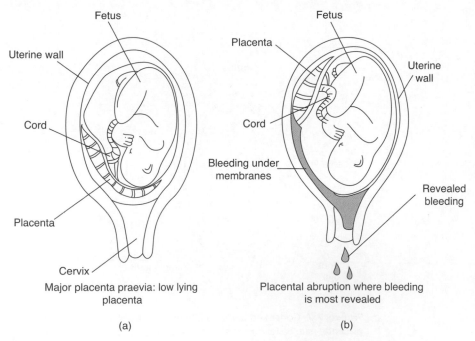

Major placenta praevia: low lying placenta

(a)

Placental abruption where bleeding is most revealed

(b)

Figure 7.3 Major placenta praevia.

occur in late pregnancy due to contractions or sexual intercourse: this causes tearing of blood vessels close to the cervical canal, commonly resulting in vaginal bleeding. Three cases of death from APH resulting from *placenta praevia* occurred between 2003 and 2005 (CEMACH 2007c) (see Fig. 7.3).

Diagnosis

The volume of revealed blood loss may be significant, particularly if the patient is in labour as this may cause further separation and tearing of blood vessels. The blood loss tends to be bright red. The uterus is relaxed and the abdomen is not tender – indeed the patient may well be pain free if they are not in labour. It should be noted, however, that the bleeding often causes uterine irritation resulting in contractions and therefore pain. Death of the fetus in utero is rare, although malpresentations are common because the low placenta prevents the head engaging in the pelvis.

As always, a thorough ABCDEFG assessment is essential. Obtaining an obstetric history is equally important: *placenta praevia* is usually identified during routine scans and patients at risk will be booked for an elective Caesarean section 14 days before their due delivery date. Recurrent episodic bleeding is common, and the patient may have already been admitted for an APH during the current pregnancy. Notably, all of the women who died from *placenta praevia* in 2000–2002 had previous Caesarean sections (CEMACH 2004).

Pre-hospital management

If the volume of blood loss is significant or the patient is in shock, **this is a time-critical emergency: rapid (lights and sirens) transportation to hospital is vital**. Follow the generic treatment guidelines for APH (see page 75).

UTERINE RUPTURE

Definition

Uterine rupture is a tear in the uterus usually associated with previous Caesarean section or other uterine surgery such as myomectomy (removal of fibroids). This is rare (incidence of 3:10,000 deliveries) and is most likely to occur during labour. It is a life-threatening emergency for mother and child.

Risk factors

- previous Caesarean section
- other uterine surgery
- grand multiparity

- undiagnosed cephalopelvic disproportion
- macrosomic fetus
- placenta percreta
- prior instrumentation of the uterus (for example surgical termination)
- external cephalic version
- uterine abnormalities (rudimentary horn)

Diagnosis
This may present with:
- if in labour:
  - ○ sudden cessation of contractions
  - ○ elevation (retraction) of the presenting part
- severe constant pain
- fetal death
- maternal shock due to concealed massive haemorrhage

Pre-hospital management
This is a time-critical life-threatening emergency requiring rapid lights and sirens transport to hospital.
Follow the generic treatment for an APH (see page 75).

PRESENTATIONS AND LIES

Introduction
It is important to understand the definitions of abnormal presentations and lies (also known as malpresentations and malpositions), and these are as follows:
- **Lie**: refers to the relationship of the long axis of the fetus to that of the mother. These are specified as **longitudinal, transverse or oblique**. If the lie changes it may be referred to as **unstable** (see Fig 7.4).

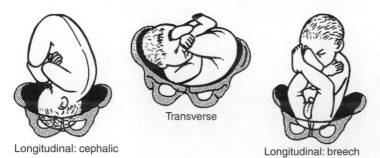

Longitudinal: cephalic   Transverse   Longitudinal: breech

Figure 7.4 Most common lies.

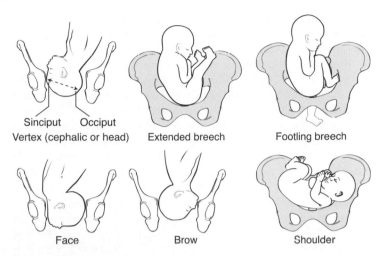

Sinciput   Occiput
Vertex (cephalic or head)   Extended breech   Footling breech

Face   Brow   Shoulder

Figure 7.5 Most common presentations.

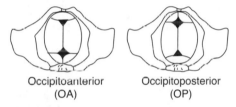

Occipitoanterior   Occipitoposterior
(OA)   (OP)

Figure 7.6 Most common positions.

- **Presentation**: refers to the part of the fetus which is presenting or foremost in the birth canal. The fetus can present by its **vertex** (also known as cephalic or head), breech (buttocks, feet or legs) **face, brow or shoulder** (see Fig 7.5).
- **Position**: refers to a reference point on the presenting part, and how it relates to the maternal pelvis. For example, the usual position is the **occipitoanterior** position (**OA** position). This occurs when the fetal occiput is directed towards the maternal symphysis, or anteriorly. However, a common malposition is the **occipitoposterior** position (**OP** position). This occurs when the occiput is directed towards the maternal spine (ALSO 2004) (see Fig. 7.6)

BREECH PRESENTATION

Definition

Breech presentation is a longitudinal lie with the fetal buttocks presenting in the birth canal, with the after-coming head in the uterine fundus (ALSO 2004; Boyle 2002). The incidence is approximately 20% at 28 weeks. However, as most fetuses turn spontaneously, the incidence at term is 3–4% (Cox and Grady 2002).

Breech presentations are associated with a higher perinatal mortality and morbidity rate, due principally to premature births, congenital malformations and birth asphyxia and trauma (Cheng and Hannah 1993; Pritchard and MacDonald 1980). Caesarean section has been suggested for breech presentations as a way of reducing the associated problems (Cheng and Hannah 1993), and in Europe and the United States, Caesarean section is the preferred mode of delivery. The Term Breech Trial suggests that delivery by Caesarean section is safer with a lower newborn morbidity for term pregnancies not in labour (Hannah 2000). As first-line management, women diagnosed antenatally with a breech presentation at term should be offered an external cephalic version (an obstetric practitioner turning the fetus by hand) (RCOG 1997). Although the management of breech presentations has changed, there will always be vaginal breech deliveries. These will occur as a result of undiagnosed breeches, rapid deliveries and patient choice. Therefore, all maternity care providers should be prepared for spontaneous breech deliveries.

Breech presentations can be classified as in Table 7.1.

Risk factors
- prematurity
- previous breech
- low-lying placenta/praevia
- pelvic masses
- bicornuate uterus

Table 7.1 Classifications of breech presentations.

	Hips	Legs	Feet	Proportion of breech presentations
Frank (extended) breech	Flexed	Extended		65%
Complete (flexed) breech	Flexed	Flexed		25%
Footling breech	One or both are extended	One or both are extended	One or both are presenting	10%

- twins or higher multiples
- polyhydramnios (too much liquor)
- oligohydramnios (too little liquor)
- fetal anomalies
- grand multiparity

Diagnosis

The signs and symptoms will be familiar to that of a normal labour and presentation. However, on inspection of the introitus the following may be visible:

- the buttocks
- feet or soles of the feet
- swollen or bruised genitalia
- meconium may be present (with the appearance of black toothpaste)

Top tip

A breech may be confused with a bald-headed baby.

Top tip

Always check with the mother if she is aware of problems like an abnormal presentation.

Top tip

Always read the patient hand-held notes. It may indicate within an alert box that this is a breech presentation.

Top tip

Assess to see if the birth is imminent, as this will affect your management.

Pre-hospital management

1 Assess the patient using the ABCDEFG primary survey, and obstetric secondary survey:

 1.1 Assess the signs of labour and determine which stage of labour the woman is in.

 1.2 Get to the point quickly and attempt to identify potential complications, such as a preterm baby, cord prolapse.

 1.3 Inform the labour ward/delivery suite of your impending arrival.

2 If your assessment indicates that you can guarantee arriving at the hospital before delivery, commence transportation without delay (lights and sirens).

Top tip

Ensure that you inform the labour ward of your impending arrival.

---

3 However, if the birth seems imminent, or you have assessed that it will occur before you reach the hospital DO NOT commence transportation:

 3.1 Request the urgent attendance of a community midwife.

 3.2 If this is a preterm breech delivery, request a second ambulance, as per management of all preterm deliveries.

 3.3 Prepare the area for a delivery; ensure neonatal resuscitation equipment is available, entonox for the mother if required, warm blankets and delivery pack.

 3.4 Support the woman in a semi-recumbent position, ensuring that her legs are supported in the lithotomy position (try using a couple of dining chairs to support the legs), alternatively the mother can support her own legs. Position her so that her buttocks are at the edge of either the bed or a sofa. The mother may alternatively choose to adopt the squatting position.

Top tip

Remember if the mother is in the squatting position, you will be behind the mother so be aware that the fetal back position may appear reversed.

 3.5 The basic principle is not to interfere with spontaneous delivery of the breech, the golden rule being the 'hands off' approach.

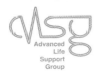

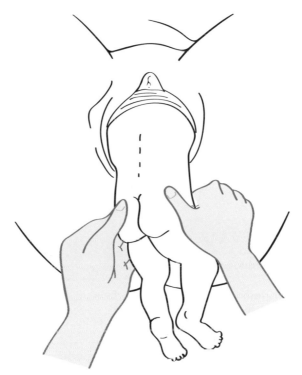

Figure 7.7 Manual rotation into sacroanterior position.

3.6 The breech will rotate spontaneously to the sacroanterior position (back anterior to the mother). If this is not the case, then gentle rotation will be necessary to achieve this position. This will involve holding the fetal buttocks over the iliac crests, and gently rotating. DO NOT hold the legs or abdomen (Fig. 7.7).

3.7 If the legs do not deliver spontaneously, they should be delivered by gentle flexion at the knee joint and abduction of the hip (Fig. 7.8).

3.8 Do NOT pull down a loop of cord.

3.9 If the arms do not deliver spontaneously, then assistance will be required using the Lovset's manoeuvre. The baby should be lifted towards the maternal symphysis and rotated until one of the shoulders is in the anterior position. Hold the baby by the pelvis – DO NOT hold the abdomen or legs. A finger should be run over the shoulder and down to the elbow to deliver the arm across the front of the body. Once the arm is delivered, the baby should then be gently rotated back to the sacroanterior position and if

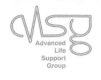

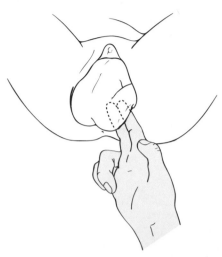

Figure 7.8 Flexion of knee and abduction of hip.

necessary the procedure repeated to deliver the other arm. Once both arms have been delivered, ensure that the baby is rotated to the original position of the back being anterior to the mother (see Fig. 7.9).

3.10 During delivery wrap a towel/cover around the baby's body to ensure warmth, but DO NOT pull on the baby.

3.11 Once the nape of the neck is visible, it may be necessary to use the adapted Mauriceau-Smellie-Veit manoeuvre, designed to promote flexion of the head, in order to deliver it. This entails supporting the trunk of the baby over your arm so that it is in the horizontal position. With this supporting arm, place two fingers into the mother's vagina, and place them on the baby's cheekbones, one on each side. With the other hand, place your index finger and fourth finger and place on each of the baby's shoulders. Pressure should be placed on the occiput via the middle finger to ensure flexion of the head. Delivery of the head should then occur by flexion of the head. Always ensure that you explain to the mother what you are doing (see Fig. 7.10).

3.12 If the baby has still not delivered, place the mother in the McRobert's position (as for shoulder dystocia) and use suprapubic pressure to aid flexion and delivery of the head.

3.13 If the head still does not deliver and the midwife has not arrived, consider the most rapid way of obtaining skilled obstetric assistance through the appropriate channels, for

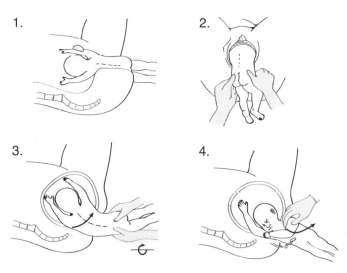

1. Here the arms are extended and cannot be delivered

2. The thumbs and fingers must grasp the baby's bony pelvis, **not** the abdomen

3. Gently flex the baby upwards ('sideways') Rotate baby 180° to bring the posterior arm to the front where it can be delivered now

4. Complete delivery of the arm Rotate the baby back 180° to deliver the second arm

Figure 7.9 Lovset's manoeuvre.

example transferring the mother to the nearest labour ward (lights and sirens)

3.14 Once delivered, assess the baby in line with standard procedures. If neonatal resuscitation is required, follow the guidelines for newborn life support (see Chapter 9).

3.15 Manage the mother post-delivery, as per guidelines for all vaginal deliveries, until the community midwife arrives.

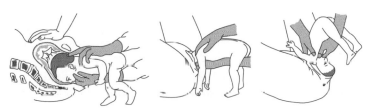

Figure 7.10 Adapted Mauriceau-Smellie-Veit manoeuvre.

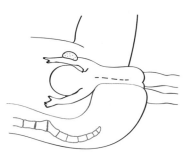

Figure 7.11 Extended head or nuchal arms.

Top tip

Pulling on the breech will complicate matters by leading to an extended head or nuchal arms, creating more difficulties and delay of the after-coming head (see Fig. 7.11).
Incorrect handling of the baby may lead to internal organ damage.

Top tip

Remember the golden rule: 'hands off the breech' whenever possible.

Top tip

Remember the fetal back must always be anterior to the mother ('tummy to mummy').

Top tip

Request the attendance of a second ambulance if this is a preterm delivery.

Top tip

Do not delay. If you are unable to deliver the head immediately assess the most rapid way to obtain skilled obstetric assistance, if no help has arrived (see Fig. 7.12)

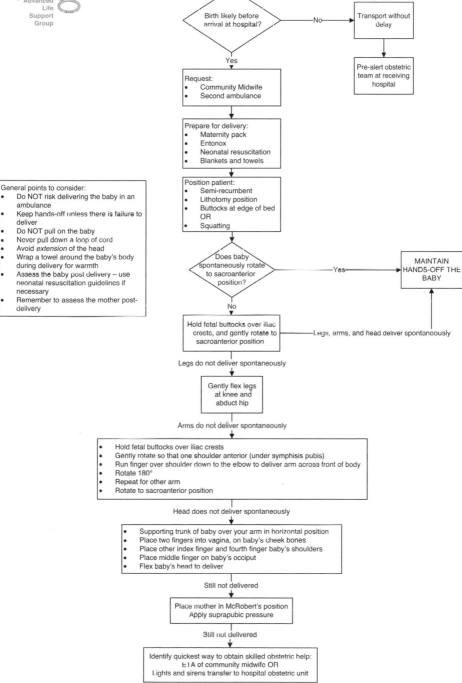

Figure 7.12 Algorithm for breech birth.

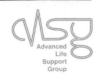
Advanced
Life
Support
Group

Occipitoposterior position

Definition
This is a malposition of the cephalic presentation. The fetus lies with its occiput towards the mother's spine. Spontaneous rotation occurs in most of these babies during labour, but fails in 5–10% of cases (ALSO 2004). Therefore, in these cases, if spontaneous vaginal delivery occurs, the fetus is born **'face to pubes'**.

The predisposing factors for an OP position are unknown, but it has been suggested that a contracted pelvis is a contributory factor (Boyle 2002).

Risk factors
- commonly adopting hip below knee posture when seated

Diagnosis
The signs and symptoms may be similar to that of a normal vaginal delivery. However, the mother may feel like pushing prior to full dilatation of the cervix, so unless you can see anything visible at the introitus, do not always assume that the mother is in the second stage of labour.

The fetal head cannot deliver until the face has cleared the symphysis pubis. Therefore, this places strain on the perineum, and these babies look like they will deliver through the rectum. Delivery of OP presentations can result in extensive perineal tearing, requiring haemorrhage control and wound repair.

Pre-hospital management
1 Manage as for all labouring women. If delivery appears imminent, DO NOT commence transportation.
2 Contact a community midwife, as for all imminent deliveries.
3 Manage as for all deliveries, but be prepared for extensive perineal tearing.
4 Once delivered, assess the baby in line with standard procedures. If neonatal resuscitation is required, follow the guidelines for newborn resuscitation (see Chapter 9).
5 Manage the mother's post-delivery, as per guidelines for all vaginal deliveries, until the community midwife arrives.

Top tip

Do not always assume that a woman is in the second stage of labour. The woman who has an OP baby may feel 'pushy' during the first stage of labour.

> A 'face to pubes' delivery may result in the mother sustaining extensive perineal lacerations, so care must be taken to assess for this.

Face presentation

Definition
This occurs in approximately 1 in 500 to 1 in 1000 deliveries (Johanson et al. 2003). The head is hyperextended so the occiput is in contact with the fetal back, and the face is the presenting part (ALSO 2004). The reference point of the fetus is the mentum, or chin.

Risk factors
- a large fetus (fetal macrosomia)
- a contracted pelvis
- enlargement of the neck caused by a cystic hygroma
- multiple coils of cord around the neck
- OP position

Diagnosis
The signs and symptoms will be similar to that of a normal labour and presentation. However, parts of the face will be seen at the introitus and can be very misleading in appearance, as the face will be very oedematous and bruised. It can be confused with a breech presentation initially. Delivery of face presentations may result in extensive perineal tearing, requiring haemorrhage control and wound repair.

Pre-hospital management
1 Manage as for all labouring women. If delivery is imminent, DO NOT commence transportation. Contact a community midwife, as for all imminent deliveries.
2 Manage as for all deliveries. The face of the fetus will sweep the perineum, and the baby will deliver, but be prepared for an oedematous and very bruised baby. Warn the mother that this will be the case.
3 Be prepared to manage extensive perineal tearing.
4 Once delivered, assess the baby in line with standard procedures. If newborn resuscitation is required, follow the guidelines (see Chapter 9). The baby born following a face presentation may have problems with its airway, due to oedema of the tongue.

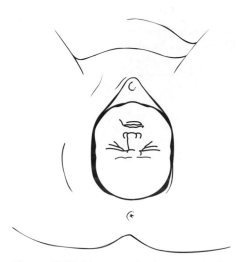

Figure 7.13 Mentoanterior face presentation.

5 Only mentoanterior face presentations will deliver vaginally. If you see a mentoposterior face presentation (eyes, nose and chin) and the baby is more than 32 weeks' gestation, then you should consider transfer as this is unlikely to deliver vaginally (see Figs. 7.13 and 7.14).

Top tip

Chin up: delivers, chin down: frown (does not deliver).

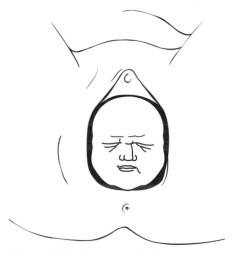

Figure 7.14 Mentoposterior face presentation.

6 Manage the mother post-delivery, as per guidelines, until the community midwife arrives.

> **Top tip**
>
> Take care not to initially confuse a face presentation with a breech presentation.
>   The mother who delivers a baby born through a face presentation may sustain extensive perineal lacerations, so care must be taken to assess for this.

Brow presentation

Definition
This is a rare presentation, approximately 1 in 5000 of all singleton deliveries (ALSO 2004). The portion of the fetal head between the orbital ridge and the anterior fontanelle presents at the pelvic inlet. The causes of this are similar to those of a face presentation. It is possible for a brow presentation to convert to a face or vertex presentation.

Risk factors
- a large fetus (fetal macrosomia)
- a contracted pelvis
- enlargement of the neck caused by a cystic hygroma
- multiple coils of cord around the neck
- OP position

Diagnosis
Diagnosis is usually only by vaginal examination, and most brow presentations cannot deliver vaginally unless they are very premature.

Pre-hospital management
Normal management is to move the mother to hospital as labour will not progress. A brow may convert to a face presentation or a vertex presentation.

Compound presentation

Definition
In this presentation, an extremity prolapses alongside the presenting part. This is usually a hand or a foot, but can on occasion be a hand and a foot. The incidence is thought to be approximately 0.04–0.14% of deliveries.

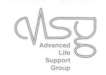

Risk factors
The causes are unknown, but it is more common in:
- preterm infants
- twins

Diagnosis
The signs and symptoms will be similar to those of a normal labour and presentation, but an extremity will be seen at the introitus.

Pre-hospital management
1 Manage as for all other types of vaginal delivery.
2 The prolapsed limb may deliver spontaneously with the head, or the fetus may retract the prolapsed limb spontaneously. If you can access the limb, flick it gently and the baby may withdraw it.
3 Warn the mother of possible bruising to the limb.
4 If the prolapsed limb is delaying descent, assess to see whether the prolapsed limb may be gently elevated upward. If not, determine the most rapid way of obtaining skilled obstetric assistance.

Transverse or oblique lie

Definition
The incidence of this is approximately 1 in 500 deliveries (Johanson et al. 2003). The long axis of mother and fetus is at right angles to each other. The fetus may lie in the transverse or oblique position, with either the head or breech in the iliac fossa. The presenting part is frequently the shoulder or cord.

Risk factors
- lax uterine muscles
- placenta praevia
- uterine anomalies
- polyhydramnios
- preterm fetus
- twins and higher multiples
- grand multiparity

Diagnosis
On abdominal palpation the uterus may feel broad, and no head or breech is found in the pelvis.

Pre-hospital management
1 In the majority of cases delivery will not be imminent; therefore, initiate transport without delay.

2 If the membranes rupture, assess for possible cord prolapse, and manage appropriately.

3 If delivery appears imminent, which may be the case in extreme prematurity (babies less than 24 weeks) DO NOT initiate transportation. Ensure that a midwife has been contacted, and manage as per vaginal deliveries.

MULTIPLE PREGNANCY

Definition

The incidence of spontaneous twin pregnancies in the UK is one in 80 (ALSO 2004).

However, the rising use of infertility treatment increases not just the rate of twin pregnancies, but the incidence of triplets and quads. The incidence of perinatal mortality and morbidity is higher in multiple than singleton pregnancies. The main cause for this is the greater frequency of premature delivery and the associated complications (Boyle 2002).

Maternal complications are common with multiple pregnancy, and these include PIH, anaemia, placental abruption, placenta praevia and PPH (Boyle 2002; Cox and Grady 2002).

Risk factors

- fertility treatment
- previous history of twins
- familial history
- multiparity

Diagnosis

Routine antenatal ultrasound scans will aid diagnosis of multiple pregnancies at an early gestation, and therefore such women will be closely monitored throughout their pregnancy. This will be documented within the woman's hand-held notes. However, if the woman has not received any antenatal care, the following may indicate an undiagnosed multiple pregnancy:

- The uterus may seem excessively large for the stage of pregnancy that the woman believes she is at (or she may deny that she is pregnant, or may actually not know).
- An excess of fetal parts may be palpated.
- If the delivery of a baby has occurred and the uterus still seems large, suspect a second fetus. This may be more evident with the delivery of a small baby from a large uterus.

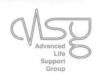

Pre-hospital management

1 Assess the patient using the ABCDEFG primary survey and obstetric secondary survey:

   1.1 Assess to see whether the woman is in labour, and if so, determine which stage of labour she is in.

   1.2 Get to the point quickly, and attempt to identify potential complications if the woman is in labour, such as:

- dealing with the possible imminent delivery of two babies which may be preterm
- dealing with possible abnormal presentations of one or both babies
- cord prolapse
- postpartum haemorrhage

Think about the other complications associated with multiple pregnancy, such as:

- pregnancy-induced hypertension
- placental abruption
- anaemia

   1.3 If your assessment indicates that you can guarantee arriving at the hospital before delivery, commence transportation without delay (lights and sirens).

   1.4 Inform the labour ward/delivery suite of your impending arrival.

Top tip

Ensure that you inform the labour ward of your impending arrival.

---

2 However, if birth seems imminent, or you have assessed that it will occur before you reach the hospital **DO NOT** commence transportation:

   2.1 Request the attendance of a community midwife.

   2.2 Request a second ambulance as there will be three (or more) patients following delivery. **There is a high chance that the babies delivered will be preterm**.

   2.3 Prepare the area for delivery. However, ensure that there are extra cord clamps, blankets and neonatal resuscitation equipment for two (or more) babies.

   2.4 Support the woman in a comfortable position for delivery – usually semi-recumbent.

   2.5 Manage the delivery as per usual guidance. Clamp and cut the first cord and await the descent of the second baby. **Do not wait long**. If there is no sign of descent of the second (or subsequent) fetus, and the community midwife has not arrived, consider the most rapid way of obtaining skilled obstetric assistance, such as transferring the mother to the nearest labour ward.

2.6 If the first and/or second twin is an abnormal presentation (for example breech), manage as per guidance.

2.7 Once delivered, assess each baby in line with standard procedures. If newborn resuscitation is required, follow the guidelines (see Chapter 9).

2.8 Manage the mother post-delivery, as per guidance for all vaginal deliveries, until the community midwife arrives.

2.9 Be prepared for PPH. Secure IV access as soon as possible.

2.10 Oxytocics should NOT be administered until the second (or final) baby has been delivered.

Top tip

Avoid giving oxytocics until the second/final baby has been delivered. **If in doubt, do not administer.**

Top tip

Be prepared for preterm babies.

Top tip

Be prepared for abnormal presentations and lies

Top tip

Do not wait long for the delivery of the second twin. Seek urgent obstetric assistance if the community midwife has not arrived.

Top tip

Be prepared for PPH.

Top tip

Beware of the possibility of multiple pregnancy in the woman who has received no antenatal care.

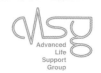

SHOULDER DYSTOCIA

Definition
A condition requiring special manoeuvres to deliver the shoulders following an unsuccessful attempt to apply downward traction. Shoulder dystocia is described as an arrest of spontaneous delivery due to impaction of the anterior shoulder against the back of the symphysis pubis. The incidence is 0.15–2% of all deliveries.

Risk factors

Antepartum
- fetal macrosomia
- maternal obesity
- diabetes
- prolonged pregnancy
- advanced maternal age
- male fetus
- excessive weight gain
- previous shoulder dystocia
- previous big baby

Intrapartum
- prolonged first stage
- prolonged second stage
- assisted delivery

> **Top tip**
>
> Remember – 50% of cases of shoulder dystocia do not have any risk factors and are associated with babies of normal birthweight (ALSO 2004).

Diagnosis
In the late second stage you may notice 'head bobbing' where the head comes forward and is visible and retracts between contractions. At delivery the 'turtle neck sign' may be seen, where the chin retracts tightly onto the perineum and the neck is not visible. Shoulders then fail to deliver with normal downward **gentle** traction.

Pre-hospital management
1 do not pull, twist or bend the baby's neck
2 do not press on the uterine fundus
3 do not cut the cord before the baby is delivered

> **Top tip**
>
> Excessive traction on the baby's neck risks significant damage to the brachial plexus.

> **Top tip**
>
> Never apply pressure to the fundus of the uterus – this will worsen impaction, may cause brachial plexus injury and rarely may result in uterine rupture.

1 Attempt to deliver the anterior shoulder with gentle downwards traction.
2 If unsuccessful after two contractions, move on to:
  2.1 McRobert's manoeuvre (in this position the pelvic diameters are increased and the angle of the pelvis is altered):
  - The mother should be asked to lie flat with only one pillow.
  - The knees should be brought up towards her chest and will abduct slightly because of the pregnant uterus.
  - Now attempt to deliver the shoulders with gentle traction downwards (see Fig. 7.15).

> **Top tip**
>
> McRobert's manoeuvre is simple and effective – about 60–70% of cases of shoulder dystocia will be managed successfully using this manoeuvre alone.

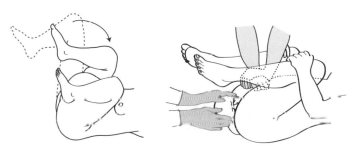

Figure 7.15 McRobert's manoeuvre.

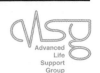

2.2 After two attempts, if the shoulders have not delivered, move on to suprapubic pressure:
- Identify the side where the fetal back lies. This will often be the opposite side to the direction the baby is facing.
- Ask whoever is helping to stand on the side of the baby's back (if the baby is facing left, stand on the mother's right or vice versa).
- Ask your assistant to use their hands in CPR grip and place the heel of their hand two finger breadths above the symphysis pubis behind the baby's shoulder.
- Ask the assistant to apply moderate pressure on the baby's shoulder pushing downwards and away from them. This will hopefully dislodge and rotate the shoulder from behind the symphysis pubis.
- The accoucheur should apply gentle traction downwards while suprapubic pressure is applied by the assistant.

2.3 After two attempts, if the shoulders have not delivered ask your assistant to apply intermittent pressure on the shoulder by rocking gently backwards and forwards:
- The accoucheur should again try two further attempts to deliver while the assistant applies rocking suprapubic pressure.

Top tip

Suprapubic pressure should be applied from BEHIND the baby's anterior shoulder – look for the back of the head and apply pressure from the same side.

---

3 After two attempts, if the shoulders have not delivered ask the mother to move into the 'all fours' position. Ensure that the mother's hips are well flexed, the bottom is elevated and her head is as low as possible (see Fig. 7.16):

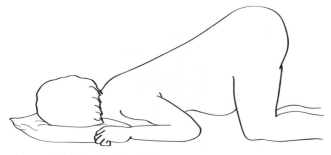

Figure 7.16 'All fours' position.

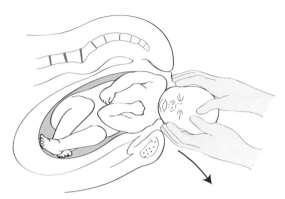

Figure 7.17 Delivery of the shoulder that is nearer the maternal back (mother in all fours position).

- In this position apply gentle traction downwards towards the floor to try and deliver the shoulder nearer the maternal back first (see Fig. 7.17).
4 **After two attempts, if the shoulders have not delivered scoop and run without further delay to the nearest staffed obstetric unit:**
    4.1 Move the mother into the ambulance, place in the 15–30° left lateral position.
    4.2 If oxygen saturation on air falls below 94% give oxygen. If SpO_2 is less than 85% use non-rebreathing mask; otherwise use a simple face mask. Aim for a target saturation of 94–98%.
    4.3 Insert one or two large-bore (14 G) cannulae on route (do NOT delay on scene to do this).
    4.4 Pre-alert the obstetric unit.

PROLAPSED UMBILICAL CORD

Definition
Prolapsed cord is defined as descent of the umbilical cord below the presenting part in association with rupture of the membranes. If it lies adjacent to the presenting part, this is known as an occult prolapse: if it is below the presenting part this is an overt prolapse. If the cord descends in front of the presenting part and before the membranes have ruptured, this is known as a cord presentation rather than prolapse. In overt prolapse the cord is displaced into the vagina and may be visible externally.

Prolapsed cord, of any type, can compromise the fetal circulation by intermittently compressing the cord between the mother and baby. This can cause fetal hypoxia, brain injury, or death, depending on the degree and duration of the compression of the cord. Over 29% of cases of overt prolapsed cord where the gestation period is less than 37 weeks will result in a perinatal death, falling to 1% if gestation is 37 weeks or more (Sethupathi 2007). Fortunately, cord prolapse is a rare phenomenon, occurring in less than 0.25% of deliveries (Uygur 2007).

Risk factors
- pre-maturity (less than 34 weeks' gestation)/low birth weight
- abnormal presentations and overt prolapse occur in
  - 0.5% cephalic and frank breech presentations
  - 5% complete breech
  - 15% footling breech
  - 20% transverse lie
- OP head positions
- pelvic tumours
- placenta praevia
- cephalopelvic disproportion
- polyhydramnios
- multiparity
- premature rupture of the membranes before presenting part engaged
- long umbilical cord (Pritchard and MacDonald 1980)

Diagnosis
Conducting a thorough patient assessment will reveal an overt cord prolapse at the introitus. Overt prolapse is most likely to be revealed at the point the membranes rupture: always examine the vaginal opening once the waters have broken. However, obtaining an adequate obstetric history will also help to raise an index of suspicion for the risk of a prolapse occurring.

Occult prolapse is normally a diagnosis of suspicion based on changes in fetal heart rate, and is therefore likely to be difficult to identify with the limited monitoring available in the pre-hospital setting. Cord presentations can only be identified by palpation of the cord within the membranes: **this is NOT a recommended intervention in the pre-hospital setting for those without formal obstetric or midwifery qualifications**.

Pre-hospital management
Overt prolapsed cord is a time-critical emergency, requiring rapid lights and sirens transfer to the nearest obstetric unit.
1 Provided delivery is not imminent, the most urgent intervention is to elevate the presenting part of the fetus above the pelvic inlet to relieve compression of the cord:
  1.1 Positioning the patient with knees to chest (face to bed) with buttocks raised is traditionally recommended for

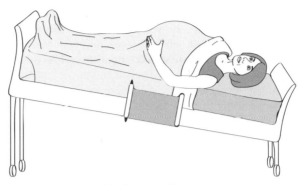

Figure 7.18 Trendelenburg position.

hospital use but is impractical and unsafe in the pre-hospital setting during transfer to the ambulance and transportation. Consequently, the mother should be placed in the 15–30° left lateral position with the hips raised by lowering the head of the ambulance trolley below the level of the pelvis (see Fig. 7.18). Remember to use seatbelts to secure the patient during transfer and transportation.

1.2 Apply manual pressure to the presenting part inside the vagina to lift it off the cord. Cradle the loop of cord gently in your palm to avoid pressing it against the vaginal wall and use the index and middle fingers to apply upward pressure to the presenting part. This pressure will need to be maintained until delivery in hospital (which is normally by Caesarean section).

1.3 As an alternative to manual pressure, a urinary catheter can be passed and the bladder filled with 500 ml of normal saline, after which the catheter is clamped until delivery. **Provided it can be achieved rapidly this should be done before moving the patient to the ambulance**.

2 Handling of the cord risks spasm and consequent fetal hypoxia. However, allowing the cord to become cool and dry will also provoke spasm, and this is a significant risk in the pre-hospital setting. Consequently, if possible, small loops of cord should be replaced in the vagina. If the loops of cord are large and replacement in the vagina is not possible, they should be covered with dressings moistened with normal saline.

3 Initiate transport using lights and sirens to the nearest obstetric unit:

3.1 Note that transfer of the patient to the ambulance can be challenging. Ideally, the trolley should be brought to the patient. If this is not practical, do NOT use a carry-chair, as this risks the mother sitting on the cord and increasing

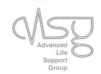

Advanced
Life
Support
Group

compression. If practical to do so and sufficient assistance is immediately available, the patient may be secured to a spine board in the 15–30° left lateral position with her hips raised on blankets. **This must NOT be allowed to delay initiation of transport**, however – if this is the case it is appropriate to bring the trolley as close to the patient as possible and ask her to walk to it.

4 Pre-alert the senior on-call obstetrician of your impending arrival.

> **Top tip**
>
> Do NOT allow your preference for preventing the patient from walking to delay initiation of transport – for example, do NOT wait for a second ambulance to arrive to assist you.

> **Top tip**
>
> If delivery is imminent encourage the woman to push actively and deliver the baby as quickly as possible. Remember to summon appropriate help as the baby may require resuscitation.

UMBILICAL CORD RUPTURE

Definition
Cord rupture is a tear in the umbilical cord. This can cause significant haemorrhage, hypovolaemic shock and even exsanguination of the fetus/newborn.

Risk factors
- short cord
- precipitous unassisted delivery (baby dangling by cord post-delivery)
- premature babies (very friable cord)

Diagnosis
Tear in the cord – you may be alerted to this by the deteriorating condition of the newborn if the tear has occurred post-delivery between the cord clamp and the baby's abdomen, or by visible blood loss.

Pre-hospital management

This is a time-critical life-threatening emergency: remember that even a small amount of blood loss from a newborn represents a significant proportion of their total circulating volume.

1 Apply direct pressure to the tear, preferably over a sterile swab.
2 If possible (that is if the tear is not too close to the abdominal wall), position a clamp proximal to the tear.
3 Whilst undertaking an ABCDEFG neonatal primary survey:
   3.1 Open, maintain and protect the airway in accordance with the patient's clinical need.
   3.2 If oxygen saturation on air falls below 94% give oxygen. If SpO$_2$ is less than 85% use non-rebreathing mask; otherwise use a simple face mask. Aim for a target saturation of 94–98%.
   3.3 Commence chest compressions if the heart rate is less than 60.
4 Based on your assessment, consider providing a bolus of 10 ml/kg of normal saline (repeated as necessary). This can be de livered via intraosseous needle, IV cannula, or umbilical vein.
5 Arrange rapid (lights and sirens) transport to the nearest hospital with appropriate facilities.
6 Pre-alert the receiving hospital.

OTHER CORD PROBLEMS

Definition

A *short cord* is defined as an umbilical cord measuring less than 40 cm. However, a cord can be:
• absolutely short – that is, its total length is limited – or
• relatively short, as might be the case with an otherwise normal-length cord being looped one or more times around the fetal neck

As the typical length of an umbilical cord is 55 cm or more, anything shorter may result in tension being placed on the cord. During labour, this can sometimes result in fetal asphyxia as the head descends. A short cord increases the risk that it will tear, resulting in life-threatening haemorrhage for the baby. Premature separation of the placenta, risking maternal haemorrhage and hypovolaemic shock for both mother and child, can also occur.

Risk factors
• no specific groups

Diagnosis

An absolutely short cord will only be diagnosed after delivery. A relatively short cord (loops) will be seen at the time of delivery of the fetal head.

Pre-hospital management of relatively short cords

Remember that this is potentially a life-threatening emergency for mother and baby.

Deliver the baby normally as most will deliver through the loops of cord. If this is not the case, you may find it easier to position the baby with the head towards the perineum until either you have unlooped the cord or it is appropriate to double clamp the cord and cut the cord between the two clamps.

Top tip

Ensure the same section of cord is double clamped before cutting.

Remember that premature placental separation may have occurred: you must therefore monitor the mother (using the ABCDEFG primary survey) for evidence of concealed or revealed bleeding and hypovolaemic shock. However, this is very rare.

If the cord is tearing or torn during or after delivery, immediately apply direct pressure to the tear and rapidly clamp and cut the cord, carefully ensuring that you clamp on both the mother and baby's side of the cord proximal to the tear – this can be challenging if you cannot visualise the whole length of the cord during delivery but failure to do so will result in catastrophic haemorrhage.

If the cord has torn, perform an ABCDEFG assessment of the newborn child. If there is evidence of significant haemorrhage or hypovolaemia, ensure bleeding at the tear is controlled by direct pressure and clamping of the cord, manage the airway, ventilate if necessary, provide chest compressions if the heart rate is less than 60 (see Chapter 9) and administer a bolus of 10 ml/kg of normal saline over 10–20 seconds (repeated if necessary).

Top tip

Avoid the temptation to routinely cut and clamp the cord if you note that it is looped around the neck. If delivery is delayed, the cord may be the baby's only supply of oxygenated blood and the baby will normally deliver through the loops.

> **Top tip**
>
> To avoid catastrophic haemorrhage if cutting the cord whilst the baby's head is at the perineum to manage a tearing/torn cord, take great care in ensuring that you clamp the cord on **both the maternal and newborn sides** proximal to the tear before cutting it.

AMNIOTIC FLUID EMBOLUS

Definition
An amniotic fluid embolus is defined as the entry into the maternal circulation of amniotic fluid, usually via the placenta. Between 2003 and 2005, seventeen such cases were reported. Ten of the seventeen babies in these pregnancies survived including one set of twins, but three of them had already delivered before the mother collapsed. The overall mortality rate in patients with suspected amniotic fluid embolus has been reported as between 26 and 61% (CEMACH 2007c).

Risk factors
- termination of pregnancy
- amniocentesis
- placental abruption and trauma
- during Caesarean section and up to 30 minutes after delivery (CEMACH 2007c)

Diagnosis
The typical scenario is one of rapid collapse in an older multiparous patient in the late stage of labour.

A clinical diagnosis is based on the triad of acute hypoxia manifested by dyspnoea, cyanosis or respiratory arrest (although initial respiratory symptoms may be minor); acute hypotension or cardiac arrest secondary to acute left ventricular failure; and coagulopathy (DIC followed rapidly by haemorrhage). Occasionally there may be premonitory symptoms up to half an hour before collapse such as feelings of doom, restlessness, altered mental status and breathlessness.

> **Top tip**
>
> Suspect amniotic fluid embolus in any patient in advanced labour with sudden collapse including hypoxia and cardiovascular compromise in the absence of any other likely diagnosis.

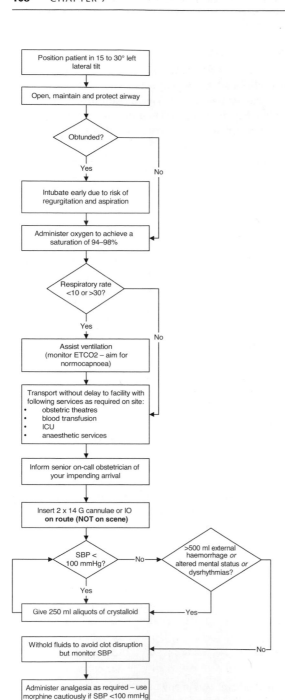

Figure 7.19 Algorithm for managing shock in late pregnancy.

Pre-hospital management

This is a time-critical life-threatening emergency requiring rapid lights and sirens transport to hospital.

Whilst performing an obstetric primary survey and obtaining an obstetric history:

1 Remember to position the mother in the 15–30° left lateral position to avoid further compromise of the fetal circulation due to vena caval compression by the uterus.

2 Open, maintain and protect the airway in accordance with the patient's clinical need. Consider early intubation in an obtunded patient due to the high risk of regurgitation and aspiration.

3 If oxygen saturation on air falls below 94% give oxygen. If SpO$_2$ is less than 85% use non-rebreathing mask; otherwise use a simple face mask. Aim for a target saturation of 94–98%. Ventilatory support may also be required. .

4 Start transportation without delay to a hospital with obstetric theatres, blood transfusion, ICU and anaesthetic services immediately available.

5 Inform the senior on-call obstetrician of your impending arrival.

6 Insert two large-bore (14 G) cannulae on route (do NOT delay on scene to do this). If it is not possible to gain IV access, consider using an intraosseous cannula.

7 Administer crystalloids in 250 ml aliquots to maintain a systolic BP of 100 mm Hg. Withhold fluids if the SBP is 100 mm Hg to reduce the risk of re-bleeding due to clot disruption unless there is evidence of significant haemorrhage, such as:
   • more than 500 ml external haemorrhage or
   • altered mental status
   • dysrhythmias

8 Administer analgesia if the patient is in pain – use morphine cautiously if the patient is hypotensive.

9 Give nothing by mouth as the patient is likely to require anaesthesia and surgery (see Fig. 7.19).

SUMMARY OF KEY POINTS

In PIH and related conditions:
• In the initial stages of pre-eclampsia, women are asymptomatic.
• Severe pre-eclampsia is often associated with headaches, visual disturbances and upper abdominal pain (right-sided).
• IV fluids must be restricted in women with pre-eclampsia because of the risk of pulmonary oedema.
• Eclamptic fits should be managed like any 'grand mal' seizure, taking particular care to protect the airway by placing in the recovery position (preferably on their left side).
• One-third of cases of eclampsia occur in the postnatal period. This is usually within 6–12 hours of delivery, but there are rare

cases in the literature, of eclampsia occurring several days post-delivery. This should always be on your differential list of diagnoses if called to see a woman in the community who has suggestive symptoms.

- Avoid administering any compound containing ergometrine as this may cause a dangerously high rise in blood pressure.

In preterm labour:

- Preterm labour is a significant predictor of neonatal morbidity and mortality.
- Abnormal presentations and prolapsed cord are more common with preterm labour.
- Preterm labour can proceed rapidly to delivery: a careful assessment may prevent the need to deliver in the back of an ambulance.
- Request the attendance of a midwife and second ambulance immediately you decide not to move a mother in preterm labour.
- Hypothermia is a particular risk for a preterm newborn.

In APH, placenta praevia and placental abruption:

- In APH, a small amount of blood lost externally can still be associated with a large concealed haemorrhage (abruption).
- Up to 30% of the maternal blood volume can be lost without a concomitant fall in blood pressure or increase in heart rate.
- Regardless of the nature of the obstetric emergency do NOT be distracted into forgetting to position a patient with a gravid uterus in the 15–30° left lateral position.
- If a patient appears to be shocked with minimal external haemorrhage and a painful tense uterus, always assume placental abruption.

In cord prolapse and other cord problems:

- Avoid the temptation to routinely cut and clamp the cord if you note that it is looped around the neck. If delivery is delayed, the cord may be the baby's only supply of oxygenated blood.
- A torn umbilical cord can result in exsanguination of the fetus/newborn and must be managed immediately.
- A patient with a prolapsed cord must be transported to an obstetrics unit without delay. DO NOT wait for additional resources to help you to move the patient.

In amniotic fluid embolus:

- Suspect amniotic fluid embolus in any patient in advanced labour with sudden collapse including hypoxia and cardiovascular compromise in the absence of any other likely diagnosis.

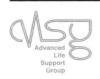
Advanced
Life
Support
Group

CHAPTER 8

Emergencies after delivery

OBJECTIVES

Having read this chapter, the practitioner should be able to define, identify and describe the pre-hospital management of:
- trauma to the birth canal
- primary postpartum haemorrhage (PPH)
- uterine inversion
- secondary PPH

TRAUMA TO THE BIRTH CANAL

Definition

Perineal trauma
This can be defined as:
- First degree, i.e. tear involving just the vaginal wall. If there is minimal bleeding, suturing is not required.
- Second degree, i.e. tear involving the perineal muscles with a corresponding tear in the vagina. Usually requires suturing, but this may be done in the woman's home by the midwife.
- Third degree includes the anal sphincter and always requires suturing in hospital.
- Fourth degree includes the anal mucosa and always requires suturing in hospital.
- Other lacerations – labial tears and grazes are common – if they are not bleeding, they do not require sutures.

Cervical trauma
- The cervix may tear if the fetus passes through an incompletely dilated cervix.
- It may be associated with other tears.

Pre-Hospital Obstetric Emergency Training, 1st edition. By Malcolm Woollard, Kim Hinshaw, Helen Simpson and Sue Wieteska. Published 2010 by Blackwell Publishing, ISBN: 978-1-4051-8475-5.

- Occasionally an obstetrician may cut the cervix in the case of head entrapment with a preterm breech delivery.

Uterine trauma

- Usually associated with previous uterine surgery such as Caesarean section or myomectomy.
- This may present postnatally with vaginal bleeding and/or shock.

Haematomas

Vulval – rupture of a vulval varix (varicose vein) or associated with perineal trauma or ruptured vulval varicosities. Can occur with a normal delivery and apparently intact perineum. An obvious painful swelling will be seen on one side of the vulva. It may present with severe buttock pain.

Vaginal – blood can accumulate in the space on either side of the vagina. There may or may not be pain and bleeding. This is a large potential space where several litres of blood may accumulate. Usually, nothing is visible on inspection of the vulva and the woman will eventually present with shock.

Broad ligament – the level of shock is out of proportion to the amount of blood loss seen.

> **Top tip**
>
> The amount of concealed haemorrhage in the case of a haematoma is often significantly greater than the volume of blood seen – be prepared to manage severe shock.

Risk factors

This can happen with any delivery, but the following groups are at particular risk:
- macrosomic baby
- assisted delivery
- shoulder dystocia

Diagnosis

- Can any tears be easily seen on the outside of the vulva?
- Is bleeding continuing despite a well-contracted uterus?
- Is there buttock pain?
- Consider whether there may be concealed haemorrhage.

Pre-hospital management

1 Gain consent and inspect the woman's vulval area.
2 If the mother is shocked, institute care as for standard management of shock and consider all causes.

3 If the mother is stable continue assessment of the vulva:

3.1 Wearing gloves gently parts the labia in order to complete your inspection.

3.2 If there is a discrete bleeding point, apply local pressure with a pad and if the bleeding is controlled await the arrival of the midwife.

3.3 Rarely, direct pressure over a bleeding point or wound will be insufficient to control haemorrhage. Under these circumstances consider the use of a haemostatic dressing – either a pad or ribbon gauze containing a haemostatic agent should be applied to the wound. N.B. Haemostatic agents should NOT be used if the wound cannot be visualised.

3.4 If a small non-bleeding tear is found await the arrival of the midwife.

Top tip

If the woman is shocked or has uncontrolled haemorrhage, treat as per PPH and move rapidly to hospital (lights and sirens).

Top tip

Haemostatic agents must **only** be used in the event that continuous direct pressure to a visible wound fails to control bleeding.

Top tip

Haemostatic agents which produce an exothermic reaction should NOT be used.

PRIMARY POSTPARTUM HAEMORRHAGE

Definition

'Primary PPH' is defined as blood loss of 500 ml or more within 24 hours of delivery and affects 3–5% of all deliveries. 'Massive PPH' is clinically more important and may be life threatening. A reasonable definition is 'loss of 50% of the blood volume within 3 hours of delivery'. Bleeding that is not so acute but continues at a rate of 150 ml/h or more, may also lead to unexpected maternal collapse. Another definition would be any bleeding that leads to haemodynamic instability. There were 14 deaths related to haemorrhage in the most recent CEMACH reporting period (2003–2005) (CEMACH 2007c). This accounted for 1 in 10 of all maternal deaths directly due to pregnancy-related causes.

Risk factors
- previous APH or PPH
- long labour
- anything that enlarges the uterus – multiple pregnancy, excess liquor (polyhydramnios), large baby
- maternal age more than 40 years
- obesity
- multiparity (especially with five deliveries or more)
- chorioamnionitis (intrauterine infection)
- known uterine fibroids
- partial separation of the placenta

The 'four Ts' is a simple tool to remind you of the common causes of primary PPH (ALSO 2004):
- tone (70%)
- trauma (20%)
- tissue (10%)
- thrombin (1%)

The commonest cause is poor uterine tone. Trauma may involve any part of the genital tract and includes tears of the vulva, vagina or cervix, as well as uterine rupture, which should be considered in cases of labour with a uterine scar (most commonly a previous Caesarean section). Tissue could mean retention of part of, or the whole placenta. Thrombin refers to the development of disseminated intravascular coagulopathy (DIC). Blood clotting mechanisms are deranged and signs include bleeding from venous puncture sites and blood that is passed does not form clots.

Diagnosis
Blood loss is notoriously difficult to estimate accurately and there is a tendency to underestimate using visible blood loss. A good 'rule of thumb' is to estimate the blood loss and then double that estimation. Maternal physiological changes include a significant increase in circulating volume which means that during pregnancy (and immediately after delivery), women do not exhibit overt warning signs of imminent collapse. In the presence of continuing bleeding, pulse and blood pressure may not change until 50% of the circulating volume has been lost. This may lead to sudden, unexpected and severe collapse and shock. If bleeding is more than expected it is recommended that adequate venous access is obtained early with two 14-G cannulae.

Although bleeding is obvious in most cases of major PPH, occasionally, hypovolaemic shock can occur without overt bleeding. In these cases, consider haemorrhage that is 'concealed' – places where significant amounts of blood can accumulate include the paravaginal tissues (a haematoma of 2 or more litres may accumulate in the tissue space) and intra-abdominally (if there has been a uterine rupture).

> **Top tip**
>
> In maternal haemorrhage, maternal collapse may not be preceded by warning signs such as rising pulse. Be prepared by gaining venous access on route to hospital with two large-bore cannulae (14 G).

> **Top tip**
>
> Not all significant PPH is visible. In the presence of shock immediately post-delivery, consider 'hidden bleeding': paravaginal haematoma, rupture of a uterine scar (intra-abdominal bleeding) and broad ligament haematoma.

Pre-hospital management

1 Fully assess ABCs – manage shock as described in Chapter 11.
2 Estimate the amount of visible bleeding (then 'double the estimate').
3 Consider causes of primary PPH (the 'four Ts') – the commonest reason is uterine atony.
4 Feel for the uterine fundus – it normally feels 'hard and firm' and just reaches the umbilicus.
5 If the uterus feels 'soft and doughy', use the hand that is holding the fundus to 'rub up' a contraction (see Box 8.1 and Fig. 8.1).
6 Give second dose of an oxytocic drug if bleeding continues (for example IM syntometrine 1 ml or misoprostol 800 microgram PR).
7 With the mother's permission, check the vulval and perineal areas for obvious tears that might be bleeding. Local compression should be applied to control bleeding.

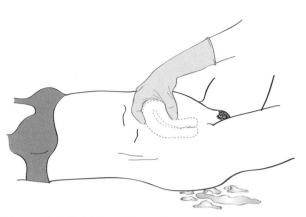

Figure 8.1 'Rubbing up' a uterine contraction.

8 If possible, consider catheterisation to empty the bladder as this will help the uterus contract.

9 If the uterus is not contracting and haemorrhage is increasing, institute bimanual uterine compression (see Box 8.2 and Fig. 8.2). This will rarely be needed but may be a life-saving manoeuvre.

10 Arrange rapid transfer to a staffed obstetric unit (lights and sirens) if bleeding continues.

11 Inform hospital about patient's condition during transfer.

12 Ask for obstetric and midwifery to be informed of your estimated arrival time.

Box 8.1: How to 'rub up' the uterus to encourage it to contract

1 Explain to the mother that this may be uncomfortable.

2 Grasp the uterine fundus firmly with your hand through the abdominal wall.

3 Gently 'massage' and 'squeeze' the uterus which will encourage it to contract.

4 During this process, blood clots may be expelled and passed vaginally.

5 If this is effective, the bleeding will reduce and the uterus will become firm to the touch and reduce in size.

6 You may need to continue this for several minutes.

7 If the uterus relaxes or bleeding continues, give an oxytocic drug.

> ### Box 8.2: How to perform bimanual uterine compression
>
> **1** This is only required if haemorrhage becomes catastrophic. It will allow control of the bleeding during rapid transfer to hospital.
> **2** Explain to the mother that this will be very uncomfortable but is lifesaving.
> **3** Use sterile gloves.
> **4** Insert two fingers into the vagina initially, then introduce the whole hand carefully and form a fist, with the back of your hand facing downwards.
> **5** Grasp the fundus of the uterus with the other hand and gently 'fold' the uterus forwards towards the pelvis.
> **6** Apply and maintain compression to the body of the uterus, between your two hands (see Fig. 8.2).

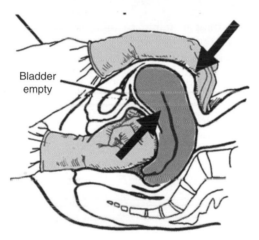

Bladder
empty

Figure 8.2 Bimanual uterine compression.

ACUTE UTERINE INVERSION

Definition

Inversion of the uterine fundus occurs in the immediate postpartum period. Inversion may be:

- 'partial' – inverted fundus remains within the body of the uterus
- 'complete' – inverted fundus protrudes through the cervix and in severe forms is visible outside the vagina

Only severe forms of inversion will be apparent in the pre-hospital setting. This is a rare complication affecting 1:2000 to 1:6400 deliveries. The commonest cause is traction on the cord without the other hand supporting the body of the uterus. Occasionally it can occur spontaneously, especially with excessive maternal pushing to try to deliver the placenta.

> **Top tip**
>
> The use of cord traction by non-obstetric practitioners is not recommended as it risks uterine inversion.

Risk factors
- associated with short umbilical cord
- associated with uterine anomalies (for example uterine septum, 'double' uterus, congenital weakness – these are all rare)

Diagnosis
Early recognition is important to minimise maternal complications. Look for the following symptoms and signs:
- severe lower abdominal pain during the third stage of labour (placental delivery)
- firm, bulging mass at the vaginal entrance (placenta may or may not be attached)
- feel the abdomen. Immediately post-delivery, the uterine fundus should be easily felt near the level of the umbilicus. In major inversion the uterus cannot be felt
- shock that is disproportionate to the amount of visible bleeding (neurogenic shock)
- shock associated with maternal bradycardia (this is due to excessive vagal stimulation because of 'traction' on the Fallopian tubes and ovaries)

> **Top tip**
>
> Consider uterine inversion in the presence of profound shock which is out of proportion to the amount of visible bleeding, particularly if there is a maternal bradycardia.

Pre-hospital management
1 Institute active resuscitation in the presence of shock.
2 If oxygen saturation on air falls below 94% give oxygen. If SpO_2 is less than 85% use non-rebreathing mask; otherwise use a simple face mask. Aim for a target saturation of 94–98%.
3 If a bulging mass is visible at or outside the vaginal entrance, an immediate attempt should be made to replace the inverted

uterus in the vagina. This simple manoeuvre may reverse the shock – see details in Box 8.3.

4 If bradycardia persists, gain intravenous access and administer atropine (500 microgram to 3 mg maximum).

5 Prepare for rapid transfer to hospital.

6 On route to hospital, ensure venous access with two large-bore cannulae (14 G).

7 Inform hospital about patient's condition during transfer.

8 Ask for obstetric and midwifery staff to be informed of your estimated arrival time.

Initial attempts to reposition the uterus in the pre-hospital situation

A single attempt at replacing the uterus within the vagina should be considered prior to transfer as this will reverse or prevent the development of shock (see Box 8.3 and Fig. 8.3).

Box 8.3: Simple manoeuvres for immediate management of uterine inversion

1 Inform patient that you are going to try to replace the womb inside the vagina and that this will be uncomfortable.

2 Ask the patient to lie on her back with her legs apart, so that you can easily reach the uterus.

3 Wear sterile gloves.

4 If the placenta is still attached DO NOT remove it.

5 Attempt to replace the uterus (and placenta if attached) back inside the vagina. Use a technique called 'taxis' [pronounced 'tax-iss']. Start by gently squeezing the part of the uterus nearest the vaginal entrance and gradually ease it back within the vagina. As the womb starts to go back inside, move your hands outwards and manipulate the rest of the uterus by gradually squeezing and pushing it inside.

6 Once the uterus is replaced in the vagina, the patient should remain lying flat. Avoid pressure on the abdomen to reduce the risk of the uterus coming back out.

7 Transfer to ambulance flat on a stretcher and maintain in this position during transfer.

8 If it is not possible to keep the patient flat after replacement of the uterus, it may be better to transfer to the ambulance first and attempt replacement there.

9 If it is not possible to replace the uterus or inversion recurs and either is associated with shock and bradycardia, remember to administer atropine 500 microgram boluses titrated to effect.

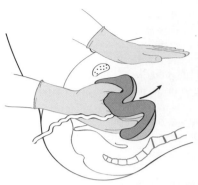

Remember to place your second hand on
the abdomen while you replace the uterus

Figure 8.3 Replacing an inverted uterus.

Additional information

The obstetric management of acute uterine inversion in hospital initially involves the manoeuvres described above. If these are
unsuccessful, the patient will be transferred to theatre and anaes-
thetised. The following options may be tried:

1 Attempt to reposition the uterus using 'taxis' under general
   anaesthesia. Once the uterus is within the vagina, the obstetrician will try to reposition the uterus by forming a 'dimple' in
   the fundus gradually pushing the womb 'outside in'.
2 If unsuccessful, 'hydrostatic' replacement is usually successful.
   This involves the obstetrician placing a hand in the vagina with
   a large-bore tube. The vaginal entrance is sealed with the other
   hand and several litres of water are introduced into the vagina.
   The vagina 'balloons' and the uterus gradually reposition itself.
3 Rarely, the abdomen will need to be opened to surgically reposition the uterus from above.

SECONDARY POSTPARTUM HAEMORRHAGE

Definition

This is bleeding that occurs more than 24 hours following delivery.
It most commonly occurs between the 5 th and 10 th day.

Risk factors

- infection
- retention of placental tissue

Diagnosis
- bleeding following delivery may have temporarily ceased or re-duced but then increases
- bleeding can be severe
- it may be associated with cramps, generalised abdominal pain and back pain
- there may be an associated pyrexia and general malaise
- the blood loss may be offensive

Pre-hospital management
- obtain a brief history of delivery and treat as per shock guide-lines
- retain any tissue that has been passed and bring to hospital

---

Top tip

Estimation of blood loss is always very difficult. Assess the degree of loss then double the figure – you are less likely to underestimate blood loss using this method.

POSTPARTUM INFECTION (PUERPERAL SEPSIS)

Definition
This is an infection in the first 4–6 weeks after delivery which usually occurs in the upper genital tract. Ten per cent of women who have been delivered by Caesarean section will develop a post-partum infection, despite being given antibiotic prophylaxis at the time of surgery. Of the women who died of sepsis 5:18 (28%) of them died in the puerperium. Sepsis was the second leading cause of direct obstetric deaths (CEMACH 2007c).

Risk factors
- infections, which are more prevalent in pregnancy such as uri-nary tract infection
- invasive procedures such as Caesarean section and instrumental deliveries
- miscarriage and/or retained products of conception
- prolonged ruptured membranes before delivery (SROM)
- chorioamnionitis
- prolonged labour
- infected haematomas
- retained swabs

Diagnosis

Infecting organisms originate from **endogenous** and **exogenous** sources. The chemicals released are:

- Endotoxins are released from gram-negative organisms typically *E. coli* and *Strep. faecalis* on their death either naturally or when killed by antibiotics.
- Exotoxins resulting from gram-positive organisms typically *Streptococci, Streptococci* and beta-haemolytic B.

Common sites of infection:

- Endometritis:
  - infection of the lining of the uterus
  - often presents with a temperature and general malaise
  - lochia may be offensive and often heavy
  - may present as a PPH
  - sometimes the focus of infection will be some retained placental tissue but often no tissue has been retained
  - rarely an abscess may develop
- Urinary tract:
  - this is a very common type of infection
  - presents with urinary frequency and dysuria
  - loin pain which may signify pyelonephritis
  - swinging temperature, sweats, fever and general malaise
  - nausea and vomiting may occur
- Wound:
  - the wound becomes red, hot and inflamed
  - there may be a hardened area above or below the wound where a haematoma has formed
  - the wound may open slightly allowing pus to drain out
  - pain can also be experienced at the wound site
  - a temperature will be present (this may be swinging) and the woman may feel generally unwell
- Perineal:
  - a tear or episiotomy site can become infected this often leads to:
    - wound break down
    - offensive lochia
    - temperature
- Other infections:
  - chest
  - viral, for example chicken pox and other childhood diseases

Pre-hospital management

1 Assess and treat ABCDEs. Treat shock as per guideline in Chapter 11.

2 **If burst abdomen:** cover the wound with a moist clean occlusive dressing and transport to hospital immediately.

3 Most other wounds should have a dry dressing applied:
  • consider assessment and treatment in the pre-hospital setting rather than transporting to hospital

4 Treatment of any infection is with antibiotics, depending on clinical condition given orally or IV. **If given orally the patient can be managed in the community with referral to GP and/or midwife.**

5 Immediate repair of the wound is usually not advisable as it will break down again.

6 Gas gangrene or necrotising fasciitis should be suspected if the wound looks necrotic or there are blisters on the skin surface. Transport to hospital for assessment.

Top tip

Check for a history of MRSA and alert the admitting hospital if previous history.

Top tip

In many cases readmission to hospital is not necessary and simple infections can be dealt with by the midwife and GP.

Top tip

DVT can present with a pyrexia of unknown origin and no other symptoms.

SEPSIS

Definition and diagnosis
For a summary of presenting clinical features, see Table 8.1.

Pre-hospital management
This should be treated as per the shock guidelines, see Chapter 11.

Table 8.1 Presenting clinical features

Infection	Sepsis
Pyrexia 37.5–38.0	Hypo-hyperthermia
Raised WCC	Low/high WCC
Site specific	Tachycardia
Pain	Tachypnoea
Uterine tenderness	Hypo-perfusion
Offensive PV loss	Oliguria
Urinary symptoms	Abnormal blood cultures
Rigors	

SUMMARY OF KEY POINTS

- The amount of concealed haemorrhage in the case of a haematoma is often significantly greater than the volume of blood seen – be prepared to manage severe shock.
- If the woman is shocked or has uncontrolled haemorrhage, treat as per PPH and move rapidly to hospital (lights and sirens).
- In maternal haemorrhage, maternal collapse may not be preceded by warning signs such as rising pulse. Be prepared by gaining venous access on route to hospital with two large-bore cannulae (14 G).
- Not all significant PPH is visible. In the presence of shock immediately post-delivery, consider 'hidden bleeding': paravaginal haematoma or rupture of a uterine scar (intra-abdominal bleeding).
- The use of cord traction by non-obstetric practitioners is not recommended as it risks uterine inversion.
- Consider uterine inversion in the presence of profound shock which is out of proportion to the amount of visible bleeding, particularly if there is a maternal bradycardia.
- Estimation of blood loss is always very difficult. Assess the degree of loss then double the figure – you are less likely to underestimate blood loss using this method.
- In cases of postpartum infection check for a history of MRSA and alert the admitting hospital if previous history.
- In many cases of postpartum infection readmission to hospital is not necessary and simple infections can be dealt with by the midwife and GP.
- DVT can present with pyrexia of unknown origin and no other symptoms.

CHAPTER 9

Care of the baby at birth

OBJECTIVES

Having read this chapter, the practitioner should be able to describe the pre-hospital management of a newly born baby at birth and identify those infants in need of resuscitation or special considerations and care. The practitioner will:

- be able to identify risk factors associated with pre-hospital delivery
- understand the difference between planned and unplanned home delivery
- describe the routine care for a term baby born outside hospital
- be able to identify those babies needing resuscitation or special care
- describe the considerations in arranging transport of the baby to hospital

BIRTH OUTSIDE A HOSPITAL SETTING

Definition

Birth outside a hospital setting may be planned or unplanned and emergency services may be called to either. If a home birth has been planned then personnel and equipment will have been organised prior to the birth. There should be plans in place for an emergency situation but such deliveries are carefully selected and at present in the UK the chances of a baby needing help at birth are less than for a hospital birth. However, for these rare events, emergency services may be asked to attend, although the lead professional is likely to remain the attending midwife. In these situations, the baby will be near term and the most likely reason to attend would be to transport a woman in labour into hospital.

Pre-Hospital Obstetric Emergency Training, 1st edition. By Malcolm Woollard, Kim Hinshaw, Helen Simpson and Sue Wieteska. Published 2010 by Blackwell Publishing, ISBN: 978-1-4051-8475-5.

Advanced
Life
Support
Group

Unplanned deliveries outside a delivery room whether at home, in an ambulance, in a shop or an emergency department are more likely to be preterm. In all these situations, it is unlikely that any emergency planning has taken place and even in an uncomplicated birth special attention should be paid to maintaining the baby's temperature.

Risk factors

- multiple pregnancies
- pregnant women involved in trauma
- women who have had previous precipitate deliveries
- concealed pregnancies (usually no antenatal care and more likely to be young or socially deprived)
- women with known risk factors for preterm delivery

Pre-hospital management

Environment and equipment outside hospital

If there is time, the equipment and environment can be prepared with a flat area for assessment and care of the baby immediately after birth. The ambient temperature should be as high as possible as maintaining the baby's temperature after birth is a priority and is more difficult outside hospital. The windows and doors should be closed to prevent draughts. Turn up the heating and obtain dry, clean warm towels for the baby at birth.

Gloves must be worn. Suitably sized equipment for airway and breathing management should be available, although the specifics will depend on local policy. Consideration must be given to clamping the umbilical cord after delivery. A clock or watch is useful to mark events and roles and responsibilities should be decided – who will take the baby and who will stay with the mother?

General care of the baby at birth

Most mature babies will breathe or cry within 90 seconds of birth and very few need resuscitation. This remains true even after precipitate deliveries out of hospital. However, every newborn baby should be assessed individually at birth and this takes place as the baby is dried. The act of drying a baby is a potent stimulus to breathe. Keeping the baby warm is essential. Due to the large surface area relative to their size they get cold quickly. At 21°C a wet baby will lose heat as fast as a naked man standing outside in the snow at 0°C. Therefore dry the baby, discard the wet towels and wrap in separate dry warm towels to avoid heat loss from evaporation or convection. Use a hat to

Advanced
Life
Support
Group

reduce heat loss from the head. If the baby is clearly well (see assessment) then he or she can be placed in direct skin-to-skin contact with the mother or other warm adult, under a warm towel or clothing.

Top tip

Wet neonates get cold quickly, particularly if preterm. Dry the baby with one cloth or towel and then wrap the baby in a separate dry towel, ensuring the head is covered.

The cord can usually be clamped about a minute after birth, keeping the baby at about the same level as the mother's uterus until this is done.

Initial assessment

At delivery collect the baby in a clean, warm towel. Whilst drying and wrapping the baby assess the condition by checking **colour, tone, breathing** and **heart rate**.

Colour: Most babies are born blue and go pink shortly afterwards. The ones in trouble are born pale or white and are more likely to need resuscitation.

Tone: This is assessed when handling the baby. Floppy babies are usually unconscious and likely to need resuscitation.

Respiration: Most babies will establish spontaneous regular breathing sufficient to maintain the heart rate above 100 beats/min and improve the skin colour within 3 minutes of birth. If apnoea or gasping persists after drying, intervention is required.

Heart rate: Auscultation at the cardiac apex is the best method to assess the heart rate. Palpating peripheral pulses is not practical and cannot be recommended. Palpation of the umbilical pulse can only be relied upon if it is >100 beats/min. A rate less than this should be checked by auscultation if possible. An initial assessment of heart rate is vital as an increase in heart rate will be the first sign of success during resuscitation.

Top tip

Auscultation at the cardiac apex is the best method to assess the heart rate.

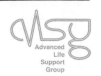

This assessment will categorise the baby into one of the three following groups:

1 Pink, regular respirations, heart rate fast (more than 100 per minute). These are healthy babies and they should be kept warm and given to their mothers.

2 Blue, irregular or inadequate respirations, heart rate slow (100 per minute or less). If gentle stimulation (such as drying) does not induce effective breathing, the head should be positioned appropriately and the airway opened. Routine suction should be avoided. If the baby responds then no further resuscitation is needed, but keep the baby warm. If there is no response, progress to lung aeration (see below).

3 Blue or pale, apnoeic, heart rate slow (less than 60 per minute) or undetectable. An apnoeic baby needs resuscitation. Open the airway and then aerate the lungs (see below). A reassessment of any heart rate response then directs further resuscitation. Reassess heart rate and respiration at regular intervals throughout.

It is important to assess the baby at birth as this guides resuscitation and a rising heart rate is often the first sign of successful resuscitation. After assessment (whilst drying and wrapping in a dry towel), resuscitation follows:

• airway
• breathing
• circulation
• with the use of drugs in a few selected cases

Top tip

As the neonatal heart is usually healthy, perinatal arrest is more likely to be respiratory. Opening the airway and appropriate aeration of the lungs will usually result in rapid improvement.

Airway

The baby should be positioned with the head in the neutral position (see Fig. 9.1).

The newborn baby's head has a large, often moulded, occiput, which tends to cause the neck to flex when the baby is supine on a flat surface. However, overextension may also collapse the newborn baby's pharyngeal airway leading to obstruction. A folded towel placed under the neck and shoulders may help to maintain the airway in a neutral position and a jaw thrust may be needed to bring the tongue forward and open the airway,

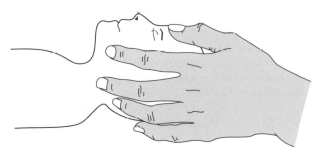

Figure 9.1 Sniffing the morning air.

especially if the baby is floppy. Visible secretions may be removed by gentle suction with a paediatric Yankauer or 12–14 Fr suction catheter, although these rarely cause airway obstruction. Blind deep pharyngeal suction should be avoided as it may cause bradycardia and laryngospasm. Suction, if it is used, should not exceed −100 mm Hg (9.8 kPa).

Breathing (aeration/inflation breaths and ventilation)

The first five breaths in term babies should be aeration (inflation) breaths in order to replace lung fluid in the alveoli with air/oxygen. These should be 2- to 3-second sustained breaths using a 500-ml paediatric self-inflating bag and a blow off valve set at 30–40 cm H_2O. Use a transparent, circular, soft mask big enough to cover the nose and mouth of the baby. It is likely that in most situations, air is as good as oxygen for resuscitation at birth. Therefore, never let the absence of oxygen delay resuscitation. Exhaled air can also be used if appropriately delivered.

The chest may not move during the first 1–3 breaths as fluid is displaced. After 5 breaths, once the chest is aerated reassess the heart rate. It is safe to assume the chest has been inflated successfully if the heart rate responds. If the heart rate has not responded, check for air entry by assessing chest movement **not** by auscultation, as in fluid-filled lungs, breath sounds may be heard without lung inflation. Confirm that the position of the head is correct; five further inflation breaths may be required to gain chest movement.

Once the chest is aerated and the heart rate has increased or the chest has been seen to move, ventilation is continued at a rate of 30–40 per minute.

> **Top tip**
>
> The FIRST FIVE BREATHS in term babies should be sustained
> aeration breaths lasting 2–3 seconds, in order to replace lung
> fluid in the alveoli with air/oxygen. A further five inflation
> breaths are sometimes required.

Circulation

If the heart rate remains slow (less than 60 per minute) after
the lungs have been aerated, chest compressions must be started.
However, the usual reason for the heart rate to remain low is that
lung inflation has not been successful – chest compressions are
rarely needed. Cardiac compromise is almost always the result of
respiratory failure and can only be effectively treated if effective
ventilation is occurring.

The most efficient way of delivering chest compressions in the
neonate is to encircle the chest with both hands, so that the fingers
lie behind the baby and the thumbs are apposed on the sternum
just below the inter-nipple line. Compress the chest briskly, **by
one-third of its depth**, giving three compressions for each ventilation breath (3:1 ratio) in the newborn (see Fig. 9.2).

The purpose of chest compression is to move oxygenated blood
or drugs to the coronary arteries in order to initiate cardiac recovery. Thus there is no point in starting chest compression before
effective lung inflation has been established. Similarly, compressions are ineffective unless interposed by ventilation breaths of
good quality. Therefore, the emphasis must be upon **good quality**

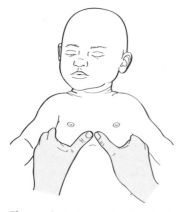

Figure 9.2 Technique for chest compressions.

breaths followed by effective compressions. Simultaneous delivery of compressions and breaths should be avoided, as this will reduce the effectiveness of both interventions.

Once the heart rate is above 60 per minute and rising, chest compression can be discontinued.

> **Top tip**
>
> Once the heart rate is above 60 per minute and rising, chest compression can be discontinued.

Drugs

If after adequate lung inflation and cardiac compression, the heart rate has not responded, drug therapy may be considered. However, the most common reason for failure of the heart rate to respond is failure to achieve lung inflation and there is **no point in** giving drugs unless the airway is open and the lungs have been inflated. Airway and breathing must be reassessed as adequate before proceeding to drug therapy. Venous access will be required via an umbilical venous line, as ideally, drugs should be given centrally. As an alternative intraosseous access may be utilised. The outcome is poor if drugs are required for resuscitation even in a hospital setting.

Adrenaline (Epinephrine): In the presence of profound unresponsive bradycardia or circulatory standstill, 10 microgram/kg (0.1 ml/kg, 1:10,000) adrenaline may be given intravenously or intra-osseously. Further doses of 10–30 microgram/kg (0.1–0.3 ml, 1:10,000) may be tried at 3- to 5-minute intervals if there is no response. For this drug the tracheal route is also accepted but effectiveness is unproven in resuscitation at birth.

Dextrose: Hypoglycaemia is a potential problem for all stressed or asphyxiated babies; however, it is unlikely in term babies at birth. It is treated using a slow bolus of 5 ml/kg of 10% dextrose intravenously, and then providing a secure intravenous dextrose infusion at a rate of 100 ml/kg/day of 10% dextrose. BM stix are not reliable in neonates when reading less than 5 mmol/l.

Fluid: Very occasionally hypovolaemia may be present because of known or suspected blood loss (antepartum haemorrhage, placenta or vasa praevia, unclamped cord) or it may be secondary to loss of vascular tone following asphyxia. Volume expansion, initially with 10 ml/kg, may be appropriate. Normal saline can be used; alternatively, Gelofusine has been used safely and if blood loss is acute and severe, non-cross-matched O-negative

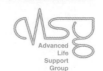

blood should be given immediately. Albumin cannot be recommended. However, most newborn or neonatal resuscitations do not require fluid unless there has been known blood loss or septicaemic shock. Excess fluid administration may complicate post-resuscitation management.

Bicarbonate: Although the administration of sodium bicarbonate forms part of the Resuscitation Council (UK) guidelines for neonatal life support, this is not routinely available in the pre-hospital setting. A Cochrane review has determined that there is no evidence of either benefit or harm for the use of sodium bicarbonate in neonatal resuscitation (Beveridge and Wilkinson 2006). If sodium bicarbonate is available, it can be given in a dose of 1 mmol/kg (2 ml/kg of 4.2% solution) intravenously (see Fig. 9.3).

Response to resuscitation

The first indication of success will be an increase in heart rate. Recovery of respiratory drive may be delayed. Babies may gasp first as they recover before starting normal respirations. Ventilation breaths should be maintained until normal breathing starts.

> **Top tip**
>
> A rising heart rate is often the first sign of successful resuscitation.

Tracheal intubation

Most babies can be resuscitated using a mask system. Swedish data suggest that if this is applied adequately, only 1:500 babies (≥2.5 kg) may actually need intubation. The technique of intubation is the same as for infants but the larynx is more anterior. This should be attempted only by personnel trained in paediatric intubation. A normal full term newborn usually needs a 3.5-mm tracheal tube, but 4.0, 3.0 and 2.5 mm tubes should also be available.

Special situations

Meconium

Meconium-stained liquor in various guises is relatively common and occurs in up to 10% of births. Happily meconium aspiration is a rare event. Meconium aspiration usually happens in term infants, when they are subject to hypoxic insult in utero before delivery. There is no advantage to suctioning the airway whilst the head is on the perineum. If the baby is vigorous, drying and wrapping in a separate towel is all that is needed. If the baby has absent

Clamp the cord, dry the baby, remove any wet or damp cloth
Cover with warm dry towels (include the head) – keep the baby warm!

↓

Initial assessment at birth
START THE CLOCK or NOTE THE TIME
EVALUATE: COLOUR, TONE, BREATHING, HEART RATE ... Do this as you dry the baby!!

↓

If not breathing ...

↓

Control the airway
Ensure head in 'NEUTRAL POSITION' (i.e. Neck is not as extended as used for opening the adult airway)

↓

Support the breathing
If not breathing – GIVE FIVE 'SLOW' INFLATION BREATHS – each 2-3 seconds duration [at 30cm H₂0]

Confirm a response – look for INCREASE IN HEART RATE and/or VISIBLE CHEST MOVEMENT

↓

If there is no response
RE-CHECK THE HEAD POSITION and APPLY JAW THRUST
REPEAT FIVE INFLATION BREATHS – use a second person (if available) to help with airway control

Confirm a response – look for INCREASE IN HEART RATE and/or VISIBLE CHEST MOVEMENT

↓

If there is still no response
A) INSPECT THE OROPHARYNX UNDER DIRECT VISION and REPEAT INFLATION BREATHS
B) INSERT A SMALL OROPHARYNGEAL (GUEDEL) AIRWAY and REPEAT INFLATION BREATHS
C) CONSIDER INTUBATION ONLY IF TRAINED IN THIS PROCEDURE IN THE NEWBORN

Confirm a response – look for INCREASE IN HEART RATE and/or VISIBLE CHEST MOVEMENT

↓

Once the chest is moving
If no spontaneous breathing – CONTINUE WITH VENTILATION BREATHS (rate 30-40 per minute)

↓

Check the heart rate
If the HEART RATE IS NOT DETECTABLE or SLOW (LESS THAN 60 BPM and NOT INCREASING)

↓

Start chest compressions
First confirm chest movement – IF NOT MOVING RETURN TO AIRWAY
APPLY THREE CHEST COMPRESSIONS TO ONE BREATH AND CONTINUE FOR 30 SECONDS

↓

Every 30 seconds Reassess Heart Rate
A) if improving STOP CARDIAC COMPRESSIONS BUT CONTINUE VENTILATIONS IF NOT BREATHING
B) if heart rate still slow – CONTINUE CHEST COMPRESSIONS AND VENTILATION (ratio 3:1)
C) CONSIDER VENOUS ACCESS AND DRUGS. CONSIDER HYPOVOLAEMIA

- AT ALL STAGES – CONSIDER USING AVAILABLE HELP
- CONSIDER WHEN TO MOVE TO HOSPITAL

Note: In the presence of meconium, remember: "Screaming babies – have an open airway"
"Floppy babies – have a look"

Figure 9.3 Resuscitation of the neonate: Newborn Life Support Algorithm, reproduced with permission from the Resuscitation Council UK, adapted for POET course October 2009.

or inadequate respirations, a heart rate <100 per minute or hypotonia, inspect the oropharynx with a laryngoscope and aspirate any particulate meconium seen using a wide-bore catheter and start mask inflation and ventilation as above. If, while attempting to clear the airway, the heart rate falls to less than 60 beats/min, then stop the airway clearance, give aeration breaths and start ventilating the baby.

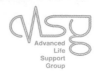

Preterm babies

Preterm babies are more likely to get cold (higher surface area to mass ratio). The more preterm a baby the less likely it is to establish adequate respirations. Preterm babies (<32 weeks) are likely to be deficient in surfactant especially after unexpected or precipitate delivery. Production is reduced by hypothermia (<35°C), hypoxia and acidosis (pH <7.25). In babies born before 32 weeks, one must anticipate a lack of surfactant. The effort of respiration will be increased although musculature will be less developed. They may require help to establish prompt aeration and ventilation and may subsequently require exogenous surfactant therapy. Many of these babies will require help with their breathing to stabilise them.

The lungs of preterm babies are more fragile than those of term babies and thus are much more susceptible to damage from overdistension. Therefore, it is appropriate to be gentle in the use of a bag, valve and mask system. Be guided by the heart rate as above.

Documentation

Actions should be documented as per normal practice. However, it is particularly useful if the following is noted:
- time of birth
- colour, tone, breathing and heart rate at birth
- time the heart rate exceeds 100 beats/min
- time of first gasp
- time when regular breathing is established
- actions taken

TRANSFER TO HOSPITAL

If only one midwife is present at a delivery then baby, mother and midwife should not be separated. If the baby required resuscitation, it will need to be admitted to a neonatal or special care baby unit. This transfer will need to be discussed with ambulance control and the receiving unit.

The ambulance heating system should be turned up to maximum. If the baby is maintaining his or her airway well, then he or she can be transported held close to his or her mother. However, if the baby requires support then special arrangements will be needed, which will depend on local practice. Some areas will use a portable incubator but the response times for such transfers are often prohibitive. It is important to know the local policies for such deliveries.

It is difficult to transfer a baby requiring active resuscitation in the same ambulance as another patient (mother). The stretcher is used as a base upon which to work but the safety of the whole team must be considered. This may be unavoidable if delivery was in the ambulance, but consideration must be given to the safe transfer of both patients.

SUMMARY OF KEY POINTS

- After drying and assessment, resuscitation at birth follows ABC.
- Temperature control, airway and breathing management will resuscitate most babies.
- If ventilation is difficult, recheck the airway position – aim to a neutral position ('sniffing the morning air').

CHAPTER 10
Management of non-obstetric emergencies

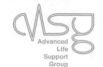

OBJECTIVES

Having read this chapter, the practitioner should be able to define, identify and describe the pre-hospital management of:
- perinatal psychiatric illness
- venous thromboembolism
- epilepsy
- diabetes
- trauma to the mother
- cardiac disease in pregnancy
- respiratory disease in pregnancy
- carbon monoxide poisoning
- rape and sexual assault in pregnancy

PERINATAL PSYCHIATRIC ILLNESS

Definition

Mental illness experienced either during pregnancy or in the post-natal period can affect not only the health but also the well-being of the mother and baby, but also those providing the usual support network around her. Mental disorders may be pre-existing or develop during pregnancy, the puerperium and up to 1 year after the birth. Practitioners should note that the term 'postnatal depression' is often used inappropriately as a general term for any perinatal mental disorder and this should be avoided (NICE 2007).

Developing a new onset of serious psychiatric illness during pregnancy is generally thought to be less of a risk than at other times, although the prevalence of all psychiatric disorders such as schizophrenia is the same in either pregnant or non-pregnant

---

Pre-Hospital Obstetric Emergency Training, 1st edition. By Malcolm Woollard, Kim Hinshaw, Helen Simpson and Sue Wieteska. Published 2010 by Blackwell Publishing, ISBN: 978-1-4051-8475-5.

women. Pregnancy itself may have a protective effect on the mother with occurrences of serious mental disorder and suicide occurring predominantly after the birth. During pregnancy, suicide rates are highest within the third trimester; 4 out of 5 deaths occurred between 34 and 40 weeks of gestation (CEMACH 2004). A summary of the incidence of perinatal psychiatric illness is shown in Table 10.1.

Table 10.1   Perinatal psychiatric illness.

Type	Incidence (2003–2005)
Suicide	37
Substance misuse	24
Medical conditions aggravated by a psychiatric disorder	18
Pre-existing psychiatric condition	15
Violence	10

Risk factors
- women in late pregnancy and the first 3 months postpartum
- previous mental health problems
- social isolation, especially if baby has been removed by social services
- previous puerperal psychosis
- recent termination
- unwanted pregnancy

Diagnosis
The pre-hospital diagnosis of psychiatric illness is difficult. Expert evaluation is always necessary. The signs and symptoms associated with psychoses or neuroses will be the same in the pregnant patient as they are for any other male or female patient. The method of suicide chosen by pregnant women is however predominantly violent in nature.

A thorough physical examination is necessary to exclude any physical cause for symptoms.

Pre-hospital management
Newly presenting psychiatric symptoms may require specific treatment such as counselling or medication. Counselling services are difficult to access in the pre-hospital environment, thus admission and referral are often essential.

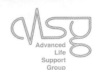

In patients presenting with a mental disorder that is affecting their health and well-being, the priority will be to provide support and guidance, not only for them but also for other family members.

It is important to assess whether the patient has the capacity to make decisions; pre-hospital practitioners need to ensure that they are familiar with guidance on gaining consent to examine or treat their patients and the focus is on the needs of the mother. If the patient refuses admission and lacks capacity they should be referred to their GP for consideration for sectioning under the Mental Health Act. Pre-hospital practitioners will have to await the arrival of other health care providers before they can leave the patient.

Referral and transfer to a facility that can provide expert evaluation is the key to the management of significant psychiatric illness; pre-hospital practitioners will need to rely on the effectiveness of their communication skills to manage these patients appropriately.

Where suicide has been attempted, the treatment and transport criteria will be the same as for any pregnant patient. Differences in treatment approaches from non-pregnant patients include:

- consideration of perimortem Caesarean section (see Chapter 11)
  - this requires very short on-scene times and lights and sirens transfer to hospital
  - notify the receiving obstetric unit
- a lower threshold for giving IV fluids
  - as with all trauma patients IV fluids should be withheld unless the patient has an SBP less than 100 mm Hg. The exceptions to this are patients with an SBP of 100 mm Hg or above and:
    - evidence of haemorrhage of more than 500 ml
    - altered mental status
    - dysrhythmias
- transporting the patient in the left lateral tilt position (15–30°)

Top tip

Remember to check that the environment is appropriate and safe for baby.

VENOUS THROMBOEMBOLISM

Definition

A venous thromboembolism (VTE) is a thrombus (blood clot) in part of the circulatory system which becomes detached. This clot is

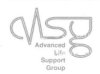

moved by the blood through the vessels and lodged in another part of the system – the location determining the severity of the symptoms. The thrombus usually originates in the deep veins of the legs or pelvis and is referred to as a deep vein thrombosis (DVT). If it is carried to the pulmonary vasculature it causes a pulmonary embolism (PE). Ileofemoral thrombi are the most common form of DVT and also are more likely to embolise. VTE is estimated to be up to 10 times more common in pregnant women than in non-pregnant women of the same age (RCOG 2001). In the period from 2003 to 2005, thromboembolism was found to be the highest direct cause of maternal death with 41 recorded cases; 33 of which were attributed to PE and 8 from cerebral venous thrombosis (CEMACH 2007c). It is predicted that many of these deaths could be avoided with improved recognition of risk factors, greater and earlier appreciation of the signs and symptoms and earlier implementation of either prophylaxis or treatment (CEMACH 2004).

Top tip

Ileofemoral DVT is more common in the left leg/pelvis in pregnancy.

Risk factors
- age (particularly over 35 years)
- obesity (body mass index greater than 30 kg/m² either pre or early pregnancy)
- parity of 4 or more
- family or previous history of thromboembolism
- gross varicose veins
- major concurrent illness (cancer, cardiorespiratory disease, inflammatory bowel disease)
- prolonged immobility, including more than 4 days of bed rest
- paraplegia
- long haul travel; this is not solely confined to air travel and includes prolonged immobility in association with car, bus or rail travel
- operative delivery; a third of all deaths from PE followed delivery by Caesarean section (CEMACH 2004)
- instrumental vaginal delivery
- prolonged labour (greater than 12 hours)
- surgical procedures in pregnancy or puerperium
- prolonged time in lithotomy

Diagnosis

The location of the embolism will determine the nature and severity of the signs and symptoms. A DVT manifests as pain and swelling in the calf muscle although lower abdominal pain may be the only presenting symptom in ileofemoral DVT. Calf tenderness, tachycardia and low-grade pyrexia suggest a DVT.

The most common findings in PE are tachypnoea, dyspnoea, rales, pleuritic chest pain, cough and haemoptysis. Clinical evidence of DVT is rarely found in patients with PE. Tachycardia may be the only sign. A massive PE may present with signs of cyanosis, hypotension, sudden collapse or death.

Top tip

Although tachypnoea, dyspnoea and leg pain are commonly found in pregnancy they should be investigated in order to exclude VTE.

The risk of VTE is as high in the first trimester as it is in late pregnancy.

Top tip

If presented with a haemodynamically unstable patient with sudden onset of tachypnoea, dyspnoea, chest pain and tachycardia, a PE should be considered in your differential diagnosis.

Top tip

Patients presenting with massive PE *may* show the following ECG changes:
- S wave in lead I
- Q wave in lead III
- T wave inversion in lead III

Pre-hospital management

This is a time-critical life-threatening emergency requiring rapid lights and sirens transport to hospital.

Whilst performing an obstetric primary survey and obtaining an obstetric history:

1 Remember to position the mother in the 15–30° left lateral position to avoid further compromise of the fetal circulation due to vena caval compression by the uterus.

2 Open, maintain and protect the airway in accordance with the patient's clinical need. Consider early intubation in an obtunded patient due to the high risk of regurgitation and aspiration.
3 If oxygen saturation on air falls below 94% give oxygen. If SpO_2 is less than 85% use non-rebreathing mask; otherwise use a simple face mask. Aim for a target saturation of 94–98%. Ventilatory support may also be required.
4 Start transportation without delay to the nearest hospital.
5 Provide a pre-alert message to the receiving hospital unit.
6 Obtain IV access on route.

EPILEPSY

Definition
This is defined as a continuing tendency to have seizures, epilepsy manifests itself through a wide range of signs and symptoms. These range from a tremor in one limb through to a whole-body convulsion, or from an unpleasant taste in the patient's mouth to unconsciousness. On average 1 in 170 people in the UK is being treated for epilepsy. It is estimated that the risk of premature death within this group is 2–3 times higher than the general population (Hanna et al. 2002).

Convulsions are predominantly classified as partial or generalised. Partial (focal) convulsions can be further subdivided as simple or complex and it is rare for either to compromise the pre-hospital patient in a way that requires immediate intervention. Generalised convulsions can also be subdivided and are referred to as either an absence or presence of a tonic-clonic episode. The latter will concern the pre-hospital practitioner in pregnancy as it can be impossible to differentiate from eclampsia. There were 11 maternal deaths from epilepsy in the period from 2003 to 2005 and of these six were sudden unexpected deaths in epilepsy (SUDEP) (CEMACH 2007c).

Risk factors
- non-concordance (poor compliance)
- sleep deprivation
- hyperemesis
- stopping anticonvulsant medication during pregnancy
- unstable epilepsy
- pre-existing epilepsy can be exacerbated by the reduced efficacy of medications through altered pharmacokinetics (caused by changes in absorption or dilution and hyperemesis)

Diagnosis
A convulsing patient may or may not have epilepsy. Most patients you are called to will be postictal by the time you arrive. A patient

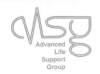

who is convulsing continuously or has a convulsion that lasts more than 5 minutes is considered to be in *status epilepticus*. It should be remembered, however, that a patient who is not known to be epileptic should be managed using eclampsia guidelines (see Chapter 7). Vasovagal attacks are common in pregnancy and may lead to generalised convulsions.

Other less common causes of convulsions during pregnancy include:
- drug or alcohol withdrawal
- pseudoepilepsy
- hypoglycaemia
- thrombotic thrombocytopenic purpura
- cerebral infarction
- hypocalcaemia
- gestational epilepsy (convulsions confined to pregnancy)
- meningitis
- cerebral vein thrombosis

A thorough ABCDEFG assessment may help identify the underlying cause of the convulsion. Getting to the point quickly is essential; this will help pinpoint the cause and the associated treatment, for instance assessing the blood glucose level and the urine for proteinuria.

Pre-hospital management

A convulsing pregnant patient represents a time-critical emergency. Whilst time at scene should be minimised, it is appropriate to stabilise your patient prior to moving her, when conditions allow.

1 The patient should be placed in the 15–30° left lateral position.
2 Open, maintain and protect the airway in accordance with the patient's clinical need, with positioning techniques, suction and adjuncts utilised as required.
3 If oxygen saturation on air falls below 94% give oxygen. If SpO_2 is less than 85% use non-rebreathing mask; otherwise use a simple face mask. Aim for a target saturation of 94–98%.
4 Rule out eclampsia – if this is not possible, treat as per eclampsia guidelines (see Chapter 7).
5 Otherwise, if the patient is still convulsing, give IV/PR diazepam (10–20 mg titrated to effect).
6 A blood glucose test should be performed; if the reading is low, the patient should be managed in accordance with the treatment of hypoglycaemia guidelines.
7 It is preferable to attempt to control the convulsion before handling and moving the patient; moving a convulsing pregnant patient is particularly challenging.

8 If the convulsion cannot be controlled in the pre-hospital environment the patient will need rapid removal to hospital. However, use sirens judiciously if you suspect eclampsia.

Top tip

Most ambulances receive patients on stretchers 'head first'. If the patient is in the 15–30° left lateral position they will be facing the wall of the saloon. Either load the patient feet first, or if this is not possible, ensure you check their airway continuously.

The important thing is moving the patient safely: this may mean moving her into the right lateral position.

DIABETES IN PREGNANCY

Definition
Patients with pre-existing diabetes are usually of type 1 (insulin-dependent diabetes). Type II (non-insulin-dependent diabetes) is increasingly common related to obesity, and may present for the first time in pregnancy. Gestational diabetes is diabetes appearing in pregnancy for the first time and can be either type I or type II. It is estimated to develop in 2–12% of women (DH 2001). It may or may not resolve post-delivery.

Diabetes is the most common pre-existing medical disorder complicating pregnancy in the UK, with approximately 1 pregnant woman in every 250 having pre-existing diabetes (CEMACH 2007a). As the diabetes epidemic proliferates, an increasing number of young people are being diagnosed.

Diabetes becomes more difficult to manage during pregnancy due to changes in physiology and metabolism. Insulin resistance increases due to the effect of placental hormones. In type I diabetes insulin requirements usually double during pregnancy. Recent studies also demonstrate that many women enter pregnancy with poor glycaemic control and half of all diabetics suffer recurrent hypoglycaemia. One in ten will become severely hypoglycaemic and require emergency treatment (CEMACH 2007a).

Normoglycaemia (4–7 mmol/l in pregnancy) is the basis of sound pregnancy care. Diabetic ketoacidosis (DKA) is rare in pregnancy. Maternal deaths from diabetes remain rare; the last triennial report for 2003–2005 indicated only one death related to diabetes (CEMACH 2007c).

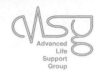

Risk factors
- obesity
- family history
- ethnic group – Indian subcontinent
- previous impaired glucose tolerance or gestational diabetes
- advanced maternal age (more than 40 years)

Diagnosis

De novo (new) gestational diabetes
- thirst
- polyuria
- weight loss
- persistent heavy glycosuria
- polyhydramnios
- fetal macrosomia
- Kussmauls respirations/DKA
- raised random blood sugar

Hypoglycaemia
This will only present in pre-existing diabetics who are receiving treatment.
- pallor
- sweaty
- malaise
- shaking shivery
- blood sugar below 4 mmol/l
- altered mental state
- reducing level of consciousness

Diabetic ketoacidosis
This is usually in association with a concurrent illness, infection (UTI is common) or poor diabetic control (sometimes due to poor concordance).
- polyuria
- nausea and vomiting
- abdominal cramps
- dehydration
- shivering
- hyperglycaemia
- altered mental state
- falling level of consciousness
- dysrhythmia
- ketotic breath
- Kussmauls respirations

> **Top tip**
>
> Hypoglycaemia and DKA in pregnancy are true medical emergencies requiring assessment and urgent hospital admission.

> **Top tip**
>
> The fetus may die as a result of poor glycaemic control. Hospital referral is important in order to check fetal well-being and viability.

Pre-hospital management

Hypoglycaemia

1 Place patient in 15–30° left lateral position.
2 Open, maintain and protect the airway in accordance with the patient's clinical need.
3 If oxygen saturation on air falls below 94% give oxygen. If SpO_2 is less than 85% use non-rebreathing mask; otherwise use a simple face mask. Aim for a target saturation of 94–98%.
4 Assess the patient's vital signs, including blood glucose level:
  4.1 if the patient is hypoglycaemic but conscious encourage the consumption of carbohydrates, sugary foods/drinks or glucose gels
  4.2 if the patient is hypoglycaemic but unconscious:
   • insert a large-bore cannula and administer 10% glucose, titrated against effect
   • if IV access is not available, give glucagon 1 mg IM
5 If the patient fails to respond, initiate transfer to the nearest hospital (not necessarily with an obstetric unit) and administer further boluses of 10% glucose titrated against effect.
6 If the patient responds, initiate transfer to the nearest obstetric unit.
7 Provide a pre-alert message to the receiving hospital.

Diabetic ketoacidosis

1 Place patient in left lateral position with 15–30° tilt.
2 Open, maintain and protect the airway in accordance with the patient's clinical need.
3 If oxygen saturation on air falls below 94% give oxygen. If SpO_2 is less than 85% use non-rebreathing mask; otherwise use a simple face mask. Aim for a target saturation of 94–98%.
4 Assess the patient's vital signs, including blood glucose level.

5 In the presence of hyperglycaemia and symptoms suggestive of DKA, do not attempt to gain IV access at scene, but initiate immediate transfer to hospital.
6 Provide a pre-alert message to the hospital.
7 On route, obtain IV access with large-bore cannulae and commence fluid therapy with a 250-ml bolus of saline repeated to a maximum of 1 L.
8 Continually monitor the patient's vital signs, with specific attention to the ECG.

TRAUMA IN PREGNANCY

Definition
Approximately 5% of maternal deaths are attributed to trauma in the UK with the majority of deaths occurring in vulnerable and socially excluded women, with domestic violence and murder being the leading causes (CEMACH 2007c). Death caused through road traffic collisions are the second largest group.

Significant thermal injury, catastrophic haemorrhage and blunt or penetrating trauma are all contributory factors in major trauma, and the cardinal rule of treatment is that resuscitation of the mother facilitates resuscitation of the fetus. In the period from 2003 to 2005, 34 women died as a result of road traffic collisions: 8 out of 21 were in moving vehicles but were not wearing seatbelts (CEMACH 2007c). Wearing the seatbelt correctly in pregnancy is now actively promoted in an attempt to reduce this trend.

Domestic violence was the recorded cause in 19 deaths in the period from 2003 to 2005 and accounted for 4.4% of all maternal deaths. Nearly all of these women were murdered by their partners (CEMACH 2004). A total of 70 out of 432 maternal deaths also had a background of domestic violence.

> **Top tip**
>
> All health care providers should be aware of the increased risk of domestic violence in pregnancy. This is often directed at the pregnant abdomen and can therefore be linked to placental abruption.

Risk factors

Road traffic collisions
• women not wearing seatbelts
• wearing the seatbelt incorrectly (see Fig. 10.1)

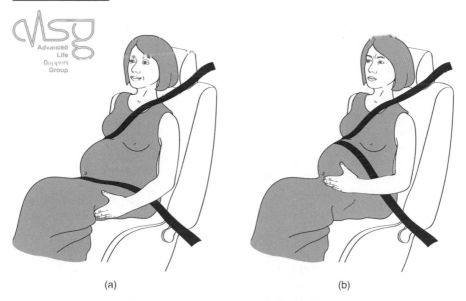

(a)   (b)

Figure 10.1   Correct (a) and incorrect (b) seatbelt wearing.

Domestic violence
- women who are in abusive relationships and/or surrounded by complex social circumstances
- young and socially excluded women
- women with children who are subject of a child protection plan
- drugs

Diagnosis
The aim is to identify injuries placing the mother and fetus at risk. Remember to consider the possibility of placental abruption (see Chapter 7). This may occur several days after the initial incident.

Top tip

Documenting the precise mechanism of injury (MOI) is imperative in the pre-hospital environment. This may aid assessment of what damage has occurred to internal organs and structures and specifically to the gravid uterus in the third trimester.

Top tip

Abruption may occur 3 or 4 days after the initial incident and after the patient has been discharged home.

Pre-hospital management

Significant blunt or penetrating trauma to the abdomen should be referred to hospital for assessment. However, most simple wounds and superficial burns may be successfully dealt with in the pre-hospital environment. A thorough ABCDEFG approach should be applied to patient assessment and ongoing monitoring. The practitioner should specifically assess for fetal movement and also ascertain if the mother is complaining of abdominal pain. The occurrence of vaginal blood loss following a traumatic incident is a red flag and should indicate that the patient is time-critical, until proven otherwise. Even significant hypovolaemia may not result in symptoms in the pregnant patient until 50% of their blood volume is lost.

1 Control any external catastrophic haemorrhage, using direct and indirect pressure or tourniquets where indicated.

2 Manually displace the uterus to the left until the patient can be secured to a spine board and tilted.

3 Open, maintain and protect the airway in accordance with the patient's clinical need, providing cervical spine protection as necessary.

4 If oxygen saturation on air falls below 94% give oxygen. If SpO_2 is less than 85% use non-rebreathing mask; otherwise use a simple face mask. Aim for a target saturation of 94–98%. Assess the efficacy of the patient's ventilation and provide assistance where indicated (persistent low saturation, inadequate tidal volume).

5 If the patient has a thoracic injury which affects the mechanism of breathing, the management and intervention must be the same as for a non-pregnant patient.

6 Disposition:
   • Any patient with a significant airway, breathing or circulation problem is time-critical and requires immediate transfer to the nearest emergency department (not necessarily one with an obstetric unit).
   • Non-time-critical pregnant patients who are injured should be taken to an emergency department with an associated obstetric unit.
   • Non-time-critical pregnant patients even if apparently uninjured should be taken to an appropriate obstetric unit for further assessment following an RTC or abdominal trauma.

7 Secure the patient onto a spine board and place sufficient padding under the right side of the board to produce a 15–30° tilt (see Fig. 10.2).

8 Insert one or two large-bore (14 G) cannulae on route (do NOT delay on scene to do this). If it is not possible to gain IV access, consider using an intraosseous cannula.

9 Administer crystalloids in 250 ml aliquots to maintain a systolic BP of 100 mm Hg. Withhold fluids if the SBP is 100 mm Hg or more to reduce the risk of re-bleeding due to clot disruption unless there is other evidence of significant haemorrhage, such as:
   - more than 500 ml external haemorrhage or
   - altered mental status
   - dysrhythmias

10 Administer analgesia if the patient is in pain – use morphine cautiously if the patient is hypotensive.

11 Apply splints to pelvic and long bone fractures.

12 If achievable, perform a 12-lead ECG and blood glucose monitoring on route.

13 Give nothing by mouth as the patient is likely to require anaesthesia and surgery.

14 If the patient has been burned assess, treat and manage their burns in exactly the same manner as for a non-pregnant patient. If burns are estimated to be more than 25% body surface area (BSA), give 1 L of crystalloid IV.

15 If the patient is non-time-critical, a full secondary survey should be performed.

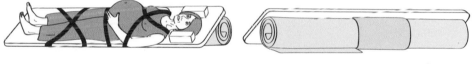

View from behind. Tilt 15–30°

(a)   (b)

Figure 10.2 Spineboard with 15–30° tilt.

> **Top tip**
>
> Remember that any pregnant patient requires hospital admission for assessment following RTC or significant abdominal trauma. The appropriate disposition is detailed in the previous section.

> **Top tip**
>
> Although abdominal and back pains are common in pregnancy, in cases of RTC and abdominal trauma, a full assessment will be required to exclude significant injury and this must be carried out in the **hospital** setting.

CARDIAC DISEASE IN PREGNANCY

Definition

Cardiac disease is generally described as congenital or acquired.

There are significant physiological changes to the cardiovascular system in pregnancy (see Chapter 3). Pregnant women with pre-existing cardiac disease may suffer an exacerbation of symptoms as a result. In the period from 2003 to 2005, 81 out of the 432 maternal deaths (18.8%) were the result of cardiac disease (CEMACH 2007c). This was the leading cause of death cited in the 2007 CEMACH report. Seventy-three deaths were related to acquired cardiac disease the most common of which was MI (16/73, 22%) followed by peripartum cardiomyopathy and sudden adult death syndrome (SADS) (12/73, 16% each). Aortic dissection accounted for 9/73 (12%) deaths from acquired disease. Congenital causes resulted in 8/81 (10%) deaths.

The rising incidence of ischaemic heart disease and obesity with an increase in average childbearing age probably account for these deaths. This is exacerbated by the increased number of asylum seekers with a childhood history of rheumatic fever, who have never had a full cardiac assessment. The incidence of non-fatal MIs is 0.6/100,000 maternities.

> **Top tip**
>
> Be aware that asylum seekers are at increased risk of cardiac disease due to an increased incidence of childhood rheumatic fever.

Risk factors
- pre-existing cardiac disease
- obesity
- Marfan's syndrome
- smoking
- family history
- diabetes
- hypertension
- hypercholesterolaemia
- maternal age over 35 years

Diagnosis

Distinguishing an acute cardiac cause for chest pain from symptoms related to gastro-oesophageal reflux (common in pregnancy) can be difficult. The practitioner must have a high index of suspicion and perform a 12-lead ECG before admitting the woman to a cardiac assessment or primary percutaneous coronary intervention unit.

It must be noted that intermittent episodes of simple arrhythmia (for example SVT or ectopic beats) are common in pregnancy and often symptoms such as palpitations do not cause significant compromise. However, a pre-hospital call to a collapsed woman where the ECG demonstrates an arrhythmia has to be construed as an emergency and should be treated as per normal guidelines and referred for cardiac assessment.

The symptoms of an acute coronary syndrome are the same during pregnancy as they are for any other patient. It should be noted that in normal pregnancy there may be some increased dyspnoea, but radiating, crushing pain is always a red flag.

Acute cardiogenic pulmonary oedema occurs rarely during pregnancy and will usually present with typical findings including coughing up pink frothy sputum, and increasing nocturnal and orthostatic dyspnoea.

> **Top tip**
>
> Aortic dissection should always be considered in pregnant women with atypical chest pain (particularly if the pain is interscapular in association with hypertension).

Pre-hospital management

Pain, acute shortness of breath or any systemic sign or symptom that compromises the patient's haemodynamic status should be considered a pre-hospital emergency. A full ABCDEFG assessment will assist in determining the nature of the problem. Remember that this is potentially a life-threatening emergency for mother and baby.

Whilst performing an obstetric primary survey and obtaining an obstetric history:

1 Manage the patient in the 15–30° left lateral tilt position or allow them to sit up.
2 Open, maintain and protect the airway in accordance with the patient's clinical need.

3 If oxygen saturation on air falls below 94% give oxygen. If SpO$_2$ is less than 85% use non-rebreathing mask; otherwise use a simple face mask. Aim for a target saturation of 94–98%.
4 If the patient is experiencing chest pain, administer 300 mg soluble aspirin to chew.
5 Administer glyceryl trinitrate (GTN) spray 400 microgram sublingually.
6 Initiate transfer to the ambulance and subsequently the nearest hospital.
7 Provide a pre-alert call to the receiving hospital.
8 Insert a large-bore cannula on route (do NOT delay on scene to do this).
9 Provide IV morphine for moderate-to-severe pain with an antiemetic if necessary.
10 Assess a full set of baseline observations, including blood glucose level and record a 12-lead ECG. **Pre-hospital thrombolysis is contraindicated in pregnancy**. However, if ST-elevation myocardial infarction has been definitively diagnosed consider taking the patient directly to a unit capable of providing primary percutaneous coronary intervention.

Top tip

Pre-hospital thrombolysis is contraindicated in pregnancy.

RESPIRATORY DISEASE IN PREGNANCY

Definition
Asthma is the most common respiratory disease in pregnancy, affecting between 4 and 12% of pregnant women (Murphy et al. 2005). The overall tidal volume in pregnancy is decreased, with an increased oxygen demand, and a mother may become breathless more easily. Asthma is associated with bronchospasm, mucosal swelling and excessive mucus production which further reduces ventilatory capacity. The severity of asthma varies, remaining stable in one-third of women, worsening in another third and improving in the remainder (Rey and Boulet 2007). In the period of the 2003–2005 CEMACH report, there were four maternal deaths attributed to asthma (CEMACH 2007c).

Tuberculosis (TB) is on the increase again, related to certain groups of immigrants and an increase in the incidence of HIV. There were two deaths from TB in the 2003–2005 CEMACH report. The incidence of TB in pregnancy, assessed by UKOSS, was 4.6 per 100,000 maternities (February 2005–August 2006).

As care with cases of cystic fibrosis has improved, more women with the disease are now becoming pregnant. These patients are more likely to suffer respiratory compromise, particularly in late pregnancy.

A woman with chickenpox (varicella) in pregnancy is at high risk of developing varicella pneumonitis, significant respiratory compromise and adult respiratory distress syndrome (ARDS).

(Also, see Chapter 10 on pulmonary embolism and Chapter 7 on amniotic fluid embolism.)

Risk factors

- women with poor asthma control prior to pregnancy
- women with a history of TB
- women with other respiratory disease
- recent immigrants/asylum seekers
- obese women
- smokers

Diagnosis

The pre-hospital diagnosis of asthma is not difficult, irrespective of whether the patient is pregnant or not. However, there is evidence to suggest that the preventative management of asthma during pregnancy is still not ideal. The differential diagnoses in pregnant women with dyspnoea will require the pre-hospital practitioner to take a full obstetric history.

Top tip

Rarely, severe pre-eclampsia may present with dyspnoea as the main symptom.

Top tip

A degree of hyperventilation is normal in early pregnancy. This should not be a concern if the patient is not distressed and there is no suspicion of more serious disease.

With significant respiratory compromise, the patient will have dyspnoea (worsened on exertion) and tachypnoea. In asthma there will be a reduced peak expiratory flow rate. They may be unable to talk in full sentences and will use accessory muscles. They may adopt a tripod posture to increase ventilation (sitting upright, leaning forwards on their arms).

Advanced
Life
Support
Group

> **Top tip**
>
> Beware the absence of wheeze in a dyspnoeic asthma patient, who is otherwise deteriorating: this is more likely to represent a significant reduction in air entry, rather than an improvement in their condition.

Pre-hospital management

The principles for the management of dyspnoea (including asthma) are the same as for non-pregnant patients. Chronic obstructive pulmonary disease is extremely rare in this group and standard high-concentration oxygen can be used in the presence of respiratory compromise. A patient demonstrating signs of life-threatening asthma should have A and B treated and should be rapidly transferred to hospital (lights and sirens).

Whilst performing an obstetric primary survey and obtaining an obstetric history:

1 Remember to position the mother in the 15–30° left lateral position to avoid further compromise of the fetal circulation due to vena caval compression by the uterus – this may need to be a semi-recumbent position if there is significant respiratory distress.
2 Open, maintain and protect the airway in accordance with the patient's clinical need.
3 If oxygen saturation on air falls below 94% give oxygen. If SpO_2 is less than 85% use non-rebreathing mask; otherwise use a simple face mask. Aim for a target saturation of 94–98%. Give ventilatory support if required.
4 Start transportation immediately to the nearest hospital for life-threatening and severe attacks of asthma.
5 For acute life-threatening and severe exacerbations of asthma, treat on route to hospital (treat on scene for moderate attacks):
  5.1 Give salbutamol 5 mg via oxygen-driven continuous nebuliser until symptoms are reversed:
    • Consider using a nebuliser attached to a t-piece and bag valve mask in patients requiring ventilatory support.
    • Salbutamol 200 microgram may be given IV only if there is no response to nebulised salbutamol in a hypoventilating patient.
  5.2 Add 500 microgram ipratropium bromide to the first dose of salbutamol for acute life-threatening or severe asthma, or in moderate exacerbations to the second nebuliser if no response to the first dose of salbutamol.

5.3 Give 200 mg hydrocortisone by slow IV push (consider oral prednisolone 60 mg for moderate and severe attacks).

5.4 If available and no response to other drugs, administer a single 1.2–2 g dose of magnesium sulphate by IV infusion over 20 minutes.

5.5 If magnesium is not available, consider 500 microgram adrenaline IM (**NOT IV**) *only as a last resort for a patient in extremis.*

5.6 Consider IV crystalloid infusion to treat dehydration and limit mucous plugging in patients having a prolonged asthma attack.

6 Transfer to hospital as lights and sirens emergency.

7 Pre-alert the receiving hospital.

8 Record a full set of baseline observations (see Table 10.2 for normal values for PEFR).

Top tip

Due to the physiological changes associated with pregnancy, overall lung capacity is reduced. Peak expiratory flow meter readings may be less than normal as predicted by the patient or a standard chart. However, in a dyspnoeic and compromised patient, treat them regardless of peak expiratory flow.

SUBSTANCE MISUSE IN PREGNANCY

Definition

The excessive use of either legal or illegal substances in pregnancy may have effects on fetal viability and growth as well as subsequent development postnatally.

Substance abuse or misuse often involves a mother either continuing to drink alcohol, smoke tobacco or cannabis, inhale solvent fumes or engaging in the use of illegal drugs such as cocaine, heroin, amphetamines or benzodiazepines. In many situations, the same individual uses more than one of the above substances at a given time. Substance misuse has a significant contribution to maternal mortality. In the CEMACH 2003–2005 report, 93 cases had problems with substance abuse; 56% of whom were registered addicts (CEMACH 2007c). The majority of drug-dependent mothers tend to use heroin as well as a mixture of other illegal drugs. The 2005 Infant Feeding Survey also reported that 17% of mothers continued to smoke during their pregnancy.

Table 10.2 Estimated PEFR ranges for women.

Age (years)	Height (cm)	Normal PEFR	Lower limit of normal PEFR	Moderate exacerbation (PEFR 50–75% best or predicted)	Acute exacerbation (PEFR 33–50% best or predicted)	Life threatening (PEFR <33% best or predicted)
15	152	385	300	193 to 289	127 to 193	<127
	160	395	310	198 to 296	130 to 198	<130
	167	400	315	200 to 300	132 to 200	<132
	175	410	325	205 to 308	135 to 204	<135
	183	420	335	210 to 315	139 to 210	<139
20	152	410	325	205 to 308	135 to 205	<135
	160	420	335	210 to 315	139 to 210	<139
	167	430	345	215 to 323	142 to 215	<142
	175	440	355	220 to 330	145 to 220	<145
	183	445	360	223 to 334	147 to 223	<147
25	152	420	335	210 to 315	139 to 210	<139
	160	430	345	215 to 323	142 to 215	<142
	167	440	355	220 to 330	145 to 220	<145
	175	450	365	225 to 338	149 to 225	<149
	183	460	375	230 to 345	152 to 230	<152

Table 10.2 (Continued).

Age (years)	Height (cm)	Normal PEFR	Lower limit of normal PEFR	Moderate exacerbation (PEFR 50–75% best or predicted)	Acute exacerbation (PEFR 33–50% best or predicted)	Life threatening (PEFR <33% best or predicted)
30	152	425	340	213 to 319	140 to 213	<140
	160	440	355	220 to 330	145 to 220	<145
	167	445	360	223 to 334	147 to 223	<147
	175	455	370	228 to 341	150 to 228	<150
	183	465	380	233 to 349	153 to 233	<153
35	152	425	340	213 to 319	140 to 213	<140
	160	435	350	218 to 326	144 to 218	<144
	167	445	360	223 to 334	147 to 223	<147
	175	455	370	228 to 341	150 to 228	<150
	183	465	380	233 to 349	153 to 233	<153
40	152	420	335	210 to 315	139 to 210	<139
	160	430	345	215 to 323	142 to 215	<142
	167	440	355	220 to 330	145 to 220	<145
	175	450	365	225 to 338	149 to 225	<149
	183	460	375	230 to 345	152 to 230	<152

(Continued)

Table 10.2 (*Continued*).

Age (years)	Height (cm)	Normal PEFR	Lower limit of normal PEFR	Moderate exacerbation (PEFR 50–75% best or predicted)	Acute exacerbation (PEFR 33–50% best or predicted)	Life threatening (PEFR <33% best or predicted)
45	**152**	410	325	205 to 308	135 to 205	<135
	160	420	335	210 to 315	139 to 210	<139
	167	430	345	215 to 323	142 to 215	<142
	175	440	355	220 to 330	145 to 220	<145
	183	450	365	225 to 338	149 to 225	<149
50	**152**	400	315	200 to 300	132 to 200	<132
	160	410	325	205 to 308	135 to 205	<135
	167	420	335	210 to 315	139 to 210	<139
	175	430	345	215 to 323	142 to 215	<142
	183	435	350	218 to 326	144 to 218	<144

Note: 'Normal' PEFR ranges may be lower in pregnant patients – the practitioner should use their clinical judgement to determine if a value below the normal ranges given above represents an acute exacerbation of asthma, based on the presence or absence of other abnormal findings. Normal values adapted from Nunn AJ Gregg I, Br Med J 1989;298;1068–70; ranges for acute asthma exacerbations based on BTS/SIGN. British Guideline on the Management of Asthma. Quick Reference Guide. London: British Thoracic Society, May 2008.

Risk factors

- socially excluded (for example being homeless or living in very poor circumstances)
- failure to access antenatal care
- other children in care or subject of a child protection plan
- history of previous substance misuse
- failure to seek or attend antenatal care

Diagnosis

A mother taking illegal substances during pregnancy increases her risk of anaemia, multiple infections (bacterial endocarditis, cellulitis and blood-borne, for example hepatitis and HIV.) The incidence of miscarriage, antepartum haemorrhage (in particular placental abruption), growth restriction and preterm labour are significantly increased when the mother has been using cocaine or heroin.

Alcohol misuse can have both fetal and maternal effects. The fetus is at risk of growth restriction and more specifically 'fetal alcohol syndrome'. Both the mother and fetus are at risk of the consequences of trauma secondary to alcohol intoxication.

Growth restriction and antepartum haemorrhage are more common amongst mothers who smoke. Miscarriage rates are more than 25% higher compared to non-smokers.

Patients who are victims of substance misuse may present with collapse and it is vitally important to exclude other obstetric and non-obstetric causes before making the assumption that collapse is due to intoxication/overdose. A history from witnesses or relatives is vital and patient hand-held records should be reviewed.

Pre hospital management

The priorities in managing a pregnant woman who is apparently intoxicated are the same as with any adult patient, other than positioning. The specific cause of collapse will dictate how the patient is managed and this is covered in other sections. General principles include:

1 The patient should be placed into the 15–30° left lateral position.
2 Open, maintain and protect the airway in accordance with the patient's clinical need, with positioning techniques, suction and adjuncts utilised as required.
3 If oxygen saturation on air falls below 94% give oxygen. If SpO_2 is less than 85% use non-rebreathing mask; otherwise use a simple face mask. Aim for a target saturation of 94–98%.
4 A full ABCDEFG assessment will assist in deciding the nature of the problem.
5 Based on the findings of your assessment, treat and manage as indicated. Remember to administer drug-specific

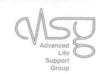

antidotes/supportive treatment if appropriate (e.g. naloxone for opiates, flumazenil for benzodiazepines, sodium bicarbonate for tricyclic anti-depressant overdose and glucagon for beta-blocker overdose).

6 Initiate transfer to the ambulance and subsequently to the nearest emergency department.

7 Provide a pre-alert call to the receiving hospital.

Top tip

Most ambulances receive patients on stretchers 'head first'. If the patient is in the 15–30° left lateral position they will be facing the wall of the saloon. Either load the patient feet first, or if this is not possible, ensure you check their airway continuously.

The important thing is moving the patient safely: this may mean moving her into the right lateral position.

CARBON MONOXIDE POISONING

Definition

Carbon monoxide (CO) occurs in the environment as a result of incomplete combustion of natural or petroleum gas. Haemoglobin has a greater affinity for CO than for oxygen. Consequently, CO molecules in the blood are readily taken up and bound to haemoglobin. This creates carboxyhaemoglobin, which is incapable of carrying oxygen, and in consequence tissue hypoxia can occur. CO is a particularly dangerous gas because it has no taste or smell and it cannot be seen.

Risk factors

About 50 people per year in the UK die at home as a result of CO poisoning through inhalation of trapped gas. Causes include faulty gas boilers and fires (in particular blocked flues and inadequate ventilation), and blocked chimneys in wood and coal burning fires and stoves. Car exhausts are a potent source of CO – fumes can build up rapidly (within minutes) in a closed garage, and whilst this can cause poisoning accidentally, it is also a method used to commit suicide.

The incidence of CO poisoning is likely to be higher in socially disadvantaged groups and the elderly, because of difficulties in the affordability of regular servicing of heating equipment.

Diagnosis

Mild CO poisoning may be misdiagnosed by the sufferer or health care professionals as a cold or flu. Symptoms may include headache, nausea, dizziness, sore throat and a cough. If it occurs as a result of a faulty house-hold appliance, it is almost certain that all family members and residents living in the accommodation will be affected – but this may increase the likelihood of a misdiagnosis of an infective cause being made.

Moderate poisoning may result in additional symptoms such as confusion, loss of memory and poor coordination.

Severe CO poisoning will cause tachycardia, arrhythmias, hyperventilation and/or dyspnoea, an altered mental status or reduced level of consciousness and convulsions. If untreated, death will ensue. The symptoms of moderate-to-severe CO poisoning may be misdiagnosed as having a cardiac, neurological or respiratory aetiology.

A differential diagnosis should be made based on the environmental evidence. Have a high index of suspicion if presented with a patient (or patients living together) with the above constellation of symptoms. As faulty heating appliances are the most common cause of CO poisoning at home, be particularly aware of this risk during cold weather when heaters have been used for prolonged periods, particularly if this occurs immediately after a warm spell or at the end of summer. If possible, ask when gas appliances were last serviced or chimneys swept.

The fire service carries CO detectors and consequently should be asked to attend any suspicious incident to assist in confirming the diagnosis.

Pulse oximetry is likely to be unreliable in CO poisoning, as most devices currently on the market are unable to distinguish between oxyhaemoglobin and carboxyhaemoglobin as they detect only two wavelengths of light. Consequently, the percentage of haemoglobin that is actually saturated with oxygen will be lower than that indicated by the SpO_2 monitor. Some newer monitors produced by the Masimo Company have the capability to measure up to seven wavelengths and this enables them to accurately distinguish between oxy- and carboxyhaemoglobin and to give measurements for both.

> **Top tip**
>
> Remember that if the mother has CO poisoning, so will the fetus.

> **Top tip**
>
> The readings obtained by most pulse oximeters are unreliable in CO poisoning: the reading provided will be falsely high and tends towards 100% regardless of the true percentage of haemoglobin saturated with oxygen. **Remember the true percentage of oxygen-saturated haemoglobin will be lower than that indicated by the SpO₂ monitor.**

Pre-hospital management

1 Consider your own safety above all else. Do NOT enter non-respirable atmospheres without appropriate equipment. If rescue is necessary, this should be performed by the fire service using self-contained breathing apparatus. If you inadvertently enter an environment contaminated with CO your only warning may be the onset of symptoms as described. If this occurs, LEAVE THE SCENE IMMEDIATELY and seek fresh air.

2 Arrange for urgent removal of the casualties from the contaminated environment – those with mild-to-moderate symptoms should be able to self-evacuate. Open windows and outside doors to allow a flow of fresh air to facilitate this.

3 Remember to place recumbent pregnant patients in either the left lateral position or tilted 15–30° to the left.

4 If necessary, secure and protect the airway: consider early intubation in severely obtunded pregnant patients.

5 If the patient is conscious, provide high-concentration oxygen, using a tightly fitted non-rebreathing mask. If the patient is unconscious and has a respiratory rate of <10 or >30, consider assisting ventilations with a self-inflating bag with an oxygen reservoir and high-concentration oxygen or a mechanical ventilator set for 100% oxygen.

6 As soon as airway access and ventilatory support have been facilitated, load and go to the nearest emergency department.

7 Provide a pre-alert message on route to the hospital.

8 Obtain IV access on route to the hospital.

9 Be aware that the patient may require urgent transfer to a facility with a hyperbaric chamber.

RAPE AND SEXUAL ASSAULT IN PREGNANCY

Definition

Rape is defined by the Sexual Offences Act 2003 as penetration by a penis of the vagina, anus or mouth of another person without

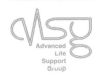

their consent. 'Consent' in the context of the offence of rape is now defined in the Act. A person can be said to have consented if he or she agrees by choice, and has the freedom and capacity to make that choice. The law does not require the victim to have resisted physically. The defendant must also show that his belief in consent of the person was reasonable. In deciding whether this belief was reasonable, a jury must consider any steps the defendant has taken to confirm that the person was consenting to sexual activity. If the victim was unconscious, drugged, abducted, or subject to threats or fear of serious harm, it will be presumed that the victim could not consent to the sexual activity and that the defendant could not have reasonably believed that the victim consented. The definition of sexual assault is similar to that of rape as the intentional sexual penetration of the vagina or anus of another person with a part of their body or anything else, where the recipient does not consent to the penetration, and the defendant cannot show a reasonable belief that consent existed (Crown Prosecution Service (March 2009))

Risk factors

Many people believe that the majority of cases of rape involve an attack on a woman by a male aggressor who is unknown to her. In reality, the majority of rape victims know their attacker. A married woman can be raped by her husband, and rape can also occur in the context of other established relationships. Victims may be raped by acquaintances or strangers. Many victims of sexual assault – perhaps the majority – do not report the offence to the police.

Diagnosis

Diagnosis should be on the basis of history. However, rape victims may be reluctant to discuss what has happened to them, perhaps because of a misplaced belief that they are in some way to blame. Consequently, pre-hospital providers must be alert to circumstantial evidence that suggests the patient may be a victim of a sexual assault. Stories of how injuries have occurred that do not match the normal mechanism of injuries found, torn clothing, a reluctance to be examined, and concerns about being left alone with male practitioners, friends, or family may all occur in the context of rape. Ultimately, the wishes of the patient must be respected, and if they do not wish to report the crime then the health care worker cannot overrule this. You should, however, tactfully try to determine the true cause of any injuries found in order that all appropriate treatment may be offered, including psychological support.

Rape is a very traumatic event. The patient may present as being confused; they may be crying, nervous and fearful, or laughing inappropriately; they may be hostile towards health care practitioners, or they may appear numb and withdrawn. Victims may delay calling for assistance, and may shower or change their clothes before doing so. In addition to psychological sequelae, signs and symptoms in pregnant rape victims may include trauma to the vagina or anus, or more general injuries resulting from the assault. Vaginal bleeding may occur subsequent to local trauma, a placenta praevia, or (rarely) an abruption. Any physical examination should be limited to that necessary to find serious injuries, and should ideally be undertaken by female health care personnel. The patient's consent to an examination should always be sought and their wishes respected.

Pre-hospital management

1 Manage the ABCs as necessary and in accordance with any injuries or illnesses found.
2 The same health care provider should stay with the patient until hand over at the hospital, once a rapport has been established. In the absence of significant physical injuries, emotional support is the most valuable intervention that pre-hospital providers can provide.
3 Although, with the patient's permission, the police should be contacted immediately, the patient should be taken to an appropriate emergency department rather than a police station. If called to the scene, the police may wish to accompany the patient in the ambulance – again this must be with the patient's agreement.
4 Remember that a crime has taken place. Even if the victim initially refuses to involve the police, try to avoid the loss of any evidence as the patient may change their mind. Tactfully encourage the victim to avoid washing, using vaginal douches, urinating, or changing their clothes to preserve evidence. Health care workers should only remove as much clothing as is necessary to safely examine the patient, and should document any damage that they have caused to clothing in doing so (for example cutting off clothes to permit access to a serious injury).
5 Carefully document any signs of trauma and any information about the circumstances of the attack that the victim shares with you. Both may be required as evidence should the victim decide to involve the police.
6 As well as treating any specific injuries or obstetric or gynaecological problems, hospital treatment will aim to determine the probability of the patient suffering a sexually transmitted

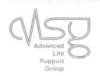

disease, and will include appropriate prophylaxis, and in planning and providing psychological support. Hospital staff may also assist the police in gathering evidence, with the patient's consent, which may include fingernail scrapings, pubic hair samples and semen as well as clothing.

SUMMARY OF KEY POINTS

- Poor medication compliance accounts for many epileptic patients suffering fits during pregnancy. Eclampsia should always be considered as a possible cause.
- Suspect a pulmonary embolism if presented with a patient with a sudden, unexplained onset of tachypnoea, dyspnoea, chest pain and tachycardia who is haemodynamically unstable.
- Good diabetic control becomes more difficult to achieve during pregnancy. This may be due to pregnancy physiology or poor concordance (compliance).
- In trauma overt signs of major haemorrhage will not be revealed until the mother has lost approaching 50% of her circulating blood volume.
- Maternal deaths from cardiac diseases accounts for more cases than all other causes together.
- In particular, acute coronary syndrome must be considered in women who are obese and/or heavy smokers.
- The severity of asthma varies, remaining stable in one-third of women, worsening in another third and improving in the remainder (Rey and Boulet 2007).
- Most incidences of acute mental disorder and suicide occur in the last trimester of pregnancy and in the first 90 days following delivery.
- The misuse of legal and illegal substances during pregnancy can have multiple adverse effects on both the mother and the fetus.
- Remember that if the mother has CO poisoning, so will the fetus.
- The readings obtained by most pulse oximeters are unreliable in CO poisoning: the reading provided will be falsely high and tends towards 100% regardless of the true percentage of haemoglobin saturated with oxygen.
- Remember the true percentage of oxygen-saturated haemoglobin will be lower than that indicated by the SpO_2 monitor.

CHAPTER 11

Cardiac arrest and shock in pregnancy

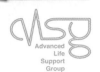

Advanced
Life
Support
Group

OBJECTIVES

Having read this chapter, the practitioner should be able to define, identify and describe the pre-hospital causes and management of:
- cardiac arrest in pregnancy
- shock in pregnancy

This chapter addresses the aetiology, identification and treatment of cardiac arrest and shock during pregnancy. As the management of adult cardiac arrest is well documented in the Resuscitation Council (UK) guidelines, which are regularly updated, this chapter discusses only those differences specific to obstetric patients.

The practitioner should also be aware of:
- the role of perimortem Caesarean section (CS)
- when perimortem CS may be considered

CARDIAC ARREST IN PREGNANCY

Principles of resuscitation during pregnancy

In general, regardless of the stage of the pregnancy, the protocols for resuscitating the obstetric patient are identical to that of any adult in cardiac arrest. However, during the third trimester some additional considerations must be made to maximise the efficacy of the resuscitation attempt and in recognition to that there being two patients involved, rather than one.

Although the fetus can tolerate quite significant levels of hypoxia, it is still reliant on the mother's body for delivery of oxygenated blood. Consequently, resuscitation of the mother should always be initiated immediately, even if her injuries appear to be un-survivable, and resuscitation should not be terminated in the

---

Pre-Hospital Obstetric Emergency Training, 1st edition. By Malcolm Woollard, Kim Hinshaw, Helen Simpson and Sue Wieteska. Published 2010 by Blackwell Publishing, ISBN: 978-1-4051-8475-5.

pre-hospital setting. This approach will maximise chances of both maternal and fetal survival.

> **Top tip**
>
> Do not withhold resuscitation or terminate maternal resuscitation attempts in the pre-hospital setting as this may compromise chances of maternal and fetal survival.

Risk factors

These groups have the greatest risk of maternal mortality (CEMACH 2004):

- Social disadvantage:
  - if both partners are unemployed, risk of maternal death is up to 20 times that of more advantaged groups
  - single mothers are more than three times as likely to die as those in stable relationships
- Poor communities – those women living in the poorest areas of England have a 45% higher mortality rate than those living in more affluent areas.
- Minority ethnic groups:
  - women from ethnic groups other than white are three times more likely to die
  - black African women (especially asylum seekers and new refugees) have difficulty accessing maternity care and have a mortality rate seven times that of white women
- Late booking/poor attendance for antenatal care – 20% of women who die book for maternity care after 22 weeks' gestation or miss more than four antenatal visits.
- Obesity – 35% of maternal deaths are in obese patients.
- Domestic violence – 14% of women who die have declared being victims of domestic violence.
- Substance abuse – 8% of women who die are substance abusers.

Pre-hospital management

Airway with positioning

Due to the risk of aortocaval compression, the patient must either be tilted 15–30° to the left (see Fig. 11.1) or the uterus must be manually lifted and supported to the left by a team member at the point that resuscitation commences (Fig. 11.2).

Failure to do so will mean that oxygenated blood cannot be circulated to the mother or fetus. Occasionally, re-positioning the uterus relative to the major blood vessels may reveal a profound syncope induced by aortocaval compression that has been misdiagnosed as a cardiac arrest.

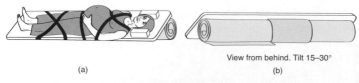

View from behind. Tilt 15–30°

(a)   (b)

Figure 11.1   Patient tilted on spine board.

Particularly during the late stages of pregnancy, the gastro-oesophageal sphincter becomes lax, gastric emptying is delayed, gastric pressure rises, and gastric fluids become more acidic, representing a significantly increased risk of regurgitation and aspiration pneumonia. Consequently, rapid escalation of airway interventions to insertion of a cuffed endotracheal (ET) tube is essential.

Top tip

In any deeply obtunded pregnant patient formal protection of the airway with a cuffed ET tube should be obtained at the earliest opportunity.

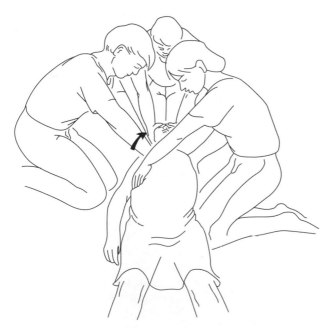

Figure 11.2   Manual tilt.

However, intubation of the trachea during the late stages of pregnancy can be particularly challenging, due to the following factors:

1 presence of full dentition
2 short obese (oedematous) neck
3 engorged breasts
4 oedema of the upper airway (if hypertensive disorders are present)
5 risk of regurgitation during intubation

Any strategy for the intubation of patients in the late stages of pregnancy must have the aim of minimising the time from commencing laryngoscopy to inflation of the tracheal tube cuff to reduce the risk of aspiration: all such interventions are, therefore, 'crash' intubations (Box 11.1).

Box 11.1: Obstetric intubation strategy

1 Remember to proceed with left lateral tilt of 15–30° applied.
2 Because of the pre-existing risk of regurgitation being exacerbated by ventilation by non-cuffed airway devices, minimise the tidal volume of ventilation via bag–valve–mask and move as quickly as possible to intubation (do not waste time attempting to hyperventilate the patient).
3 Have suction running with the tip placed under the patient's shoulder. Use wide-bore tubing, not an ET catheter.
4 Prepare the ET tube for a crash intubation: cut to length, and with a syringe, catheter mount, and tube-tie pre-attached.
5 Prepare a second ET tube one size smaller than normal, as above. This may be required in the event of laryngeal oedema.
6 Prepare an ET tube introducer (bougie) for use, curving the bougie and ensuring the distal tip is formed into a J (coudé) shape. **Always use a bougie in the pre-hospital setting.**
7 Consider using a number four laryngoscope blade.
8 Use at least one pillow or equivalent to place the patient's head in the 'sniffing the morning air' position (unless suspicion of cervical-spine trauma).
9 Insertion of the laryngoscope may prove very difficult in pregnant patients. This may be overcome by removing the blade from the handle, inserting it, and then re-attaching the handle with the blade in the mouth.
10 Since there is a high risk of regurgitation, an assistant should apply Sellick's manoeuvre. This differs from cricothyroid pressure in that a hand must be placed under the neck as well as on the cricoid cartilage. This action helps to compress the oesophagus

Box 11.1: Obstetric intubation strategy (continued)

to minimise the risk of regurgitation, and has the additional benefit of bringing an anterior glottis into view. **Sellick's manoeuvre must not be discontinued until the ET tube has been correctly positioned and the cuff inflated**.

11 Perform a laryngoscopy, obtaining the best possible view of the glottic opening.

   11.1 You should always be able to view the tip of the epiglottis and, ideally, the arytenoid cartilages.

   11.2 Advance the bougie in the midline, continually observing its distal tip, with the concavity facing anteriorly.

   11.3 Visualise the tip of the bougie passing posterior to the epiglottis and (where possible) anterior to the arytenoid cartilages.

   11.4 Once the tip of the bougie has passed the epiglottis, continue to advance it in the midline so that it passes behind the epiglottis but in an anterior direction.

   11.5 As the tip of the bougie enters the glottic opening you will either feel 'clicks' as it passes over the tracheal rings or the tip will arrest against the wall of the airways ('hold-up'). This suggests correct insertion, although cannot be relied upon to indicate correct positioning with 100% accuracy. **However, failure to elicit clicks or hold-up is indicative of oesophageal placement**.

   11.6 Hold the bougie firmly in place **and maintain laryngoscopy**.

      11.6.1 Instruct a colleague to pass the ET tube over the proximal end of the bougie.

      11.6.2 As the proximal tip of the bougie is re-exposed, the assistant should carefully grasp it, assuming control of the bougie and passing control of the ET tube to the intubator.

      11.6.3 The ET tube should then be carefully advanced ('rail-roaded') along the bougie and hence through the glottic opening, taking care to avoid movement of the bougie.

      11.6.4 Successful intubation may be considerably enhanced by rotating the ET tube 90° anti-clockwise, so that the bevel faces posteriorly. In so doing the bougie will also rotate along the same plane but should not be allowed to move up or down the trachea.

   11.7 Once the ET tube is fully in place, hold it securely as your colleague withdraws the bougie.

   11.8 Withdraw the laryngoscope.

Box 11.1: Obstetric intubation strategy (continued)

12 Inflate the cuff without delay. Then verify correct positioning of the ET tube using auscultation of the lung fields and epigastrium and observing for chest wall movement.

13 Tie the tube securely into place. The tip of the ET tube can move up to 6.0 cm once placed and this is certainly sufficient to dislodge it from the trachea.

14 Re-confirm tube placement using an oesophageal detector device (Fig. 11.3) and continuous quantitative waveform end-tidal CO_2 monitoring. Re-check every time the patient is moved.

15 Position an appropriately sized oropharyngeal airway alongside the ET tube to serve as a bite block should the patient's level of consciousness change.

16 Each intubation attempt must take no more than 30 seconds from the point at which the last inflation is given to the time at which the first inflation is delivered via the tracheal tube. After 20 seconds has expired, if the tracheal tube has not been passed through the vocal cords, abandon the procedure and consider whether someone else in the team is more likely to be successful. If not, abandon tracheal intubation and use a laryngeal mask airway (LMA), carefully monitoring for evidence of regurgitation. If ventilation is not possible or regurgitation occurs (gastric contents in the LMA) move to surgical cricothyroidotomy. Note that no more than a total of two intubation attempts is appropriate before using other means to manage the airway.

Tracheal intubation with a cuffed tube is the gold standard of airway management, and this is particularly true in the obstetric patient due to the increased risk of regurgitation and aspiration of highly acidic stomach contents. However, it is a challenging

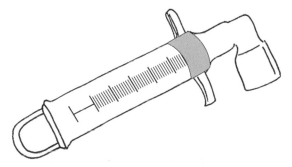

Figure 11.3 Oesophageal detector device.

procedure, particularly in third trimester patients. Consequently, if it proves impossible to perform, alternative interventions should be considered.

Laryngeal mask airway

Insertion of an LMA is performed without the need to visualise the glottis and it requires less skill to use than a tracheal tube; indeed, it is increasingly being utilised by basic-life support level practitioners. It is considered to be safer and more effective than naso- or oropharyngeal airways, producing less gastric distension during positive-pressure ventilation and reducing the probability of regurgitation. However, if regurgitation does occur, a standard LMA is less effective than a tracheal tube at preventing aspiration. Further, the seal at the glottic opening is relatively weak and permits only low pressures to be used during ventilation: this can be a particular problem in late pregnancy as the chest wall is less compliant than normal and the lungs are splinted by the high diaphragm. Consequently, the LMA should only be used in obstetric patients if intubation skills are not available or intubation attempts have failed.

A newer LMA design called the Proseal is more effective at limiting aspiration and permitting higher ventilation pressures. It has an additional posterior cuff to push the distal opening of the LMA more securely over the glottic opening and the facility to pass a small gastric tube to facilitate decompression of the stomach. A disposable version is now available.

Combitube

The Combitube is a double-lumen device that, like the LMA, is designed to be inserted blind without the need to visualise the glottis. In addition to permitting positive-pressure ventilation it is effective at preventing aspiration due to its distal and proximal cuff design. Ventilation is performed either via openings in a short hypopharyngeal tube (most commonly) or occasionally via a long cuffed tube sited in the trachea, depending on where the longer tube is sited following insertion.

There have been infrequent reports of oesophageal trauma (approximately 3 per 1000 cases) following use of the Combitube and it can only be used in patients over 5 ft tall. Unfortunately, there is little experience of Combitube use in the UK, and it has not, therefore, been widely adopted outside the USA.

Breathing

As described previously, ventilation with a bag–valve–mask should be avoided due to the increased risk of gastric distension during positive-pressure ventilation and subsequent regurgitation and aspiration. Further, the decreased compliance of the chest wall and splinting of the lungs by the diaphragm makes lung expansion much more difficult to achieve and requires higher pressures to facilitate, again increasing the risk of gastric distension, regurgitation and aspiration. Consequently, ventilation should be provided via some form of cuffed airway device (ET tube, LMA, Combitube, or surgical cricothyroidotomy as a last resort).

Due to the increased metabolic requirement in pregnancy, the highest possible concentration of oxygen should be administered during ventilation, using an appropriate reservoir bag or automatic ventilator. To avoid cerebral vasoconstriction or vasodilation in mother and fetus, normocapneoa must be maintained and this is best facilitated by using an automatic ventilator in conjunction with waveform end-tidal CO_2 monitoring to set an appropriate rate and tidal volume.

> **Top tip**
>
> Ventilation of the pregnant patient with a bag–valve–mask and naso- or oropharyngeal airway is unwise due to the significant risk of regurgitation and aspiration. Instead, a cuffed device (ET tube, LMA, or Combitube) should be used.

Circulation

Chest compressions administered to a supine patient in the third trimester of pregnancy are unlikely to result in an adequate cardiac output due to the effects of aortocaval compression. As a brief intervention until help is available, a lone practitioner can position himself or herself to perform chest compressions with his or her knees under the patient's right chest wall with the aim of tilting them to the left to re-position the uterus.

As soon as possible (and as one of the first interventions to be performed when the required equipment is available) the patient should be strapped to a long spine board which should then be tilted 15–30° to the left. This should be supported in position using non-compressible materials such as tightly rolled blankets. This will also provide a firm surface against which to perform chest compressions. The head blocks must be used to prevent malpositioning of the patient's airway under the effects of gravity (see Fig. 11.1). If further help arrives without a spine board, one member of the team must be permanently assigned to manually displace the uterus to the left.

> **Top tip**
>
> Chest compressions administered to a supine patient in the third trimester of pregnancy are unlikely to result in an adequate cardiac output.

In other respects, the procedures and advanced life support protocols for managing cardiac arrest are the same for the pregnant patient as they are for any adult (Fig. 11.4). Ventilation to compression ratios, defibrillator electrode position and energy settings and drug doses are all unaltered. However, if cardiac arrest is refractory to the completion of a second loop of 2 minutes of 30:2 CPR (second set of five cycles of 30:2), the patient should be transported immediately with ongoing CPR to the nearest hospital with full obstetric theatre facilities to facilitate emergency Caesarean section (CS). CPR should *not* be terminated in the pre-hospital setting, even if the prognosis for the mother is poor, as the fetus may still survive. Any delays or pauses in CPR will significantly reduce the probability of survival of both the mother and the fetus.

> **Top tip**
>
> The most common presenting cardiac arrest rhythm in pregnancy is pulseless electrical activity (PEA).

As with victims of trauma, the treatment of cardiac arrest secondary to haemorrhage requires rapid surgical intervention in the pregnant patient. Indeed, if any patient after 24 weeks' pregnancy fails to respond to 4 minutes of active CPR, the aim is to perform a perimortem CS as soon as possible. Consequently, in all such cases the patient should be positioned on a spine board with 15–30° left lateral tilt. Their airway should be secured and urgent transport initiated, with ongoing CPR to the nearest emergency department with senior obstetric staff available on site. There should be no delay on scene to cannulate the patient: rather this should be performed on route to hospital and IV crystalloids given in 250 ml aliquots to maintain a systolic BP of 100 mm Hg. Withhold fluids if the SBP is 100 mm Hg or above to reduce the risk of re-bleeding due to clot disruption unless there is other evidence of significant haemorrhage, such as:
- more than 500 ml external haemorrhage or
- altered mental status
- dysrhythmias

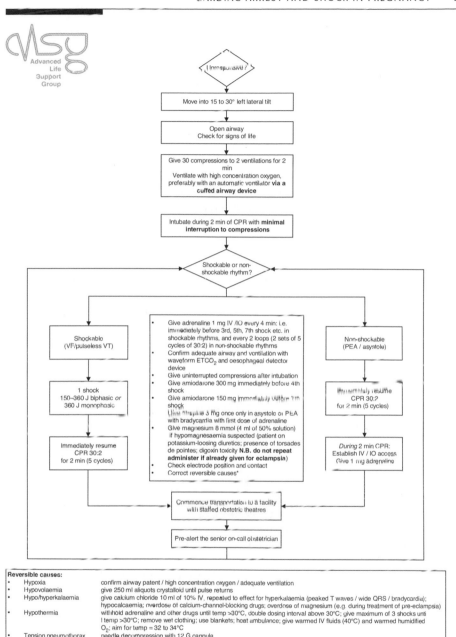

Reversible causes:

• Hypoxia	confirm airway patent / high concentration oxygen / adequate ventilation
• Hypovolaemia	give 250 ml aliquots crystalloid until pulse returns
• Hypo/hyperkalaemia	give calcium chloride 10 ml of 10% IV, repeated to effect for hyperkalaemia (peaked T waves / wide QRS / bradycardia); hypocalcaemia; overdose of calcium-channel-blocking drugs; overdose of magnesium (e.g. during treatment of pre-eclampsia)
• Hypothermia	withhold adrenaline and other drugs until temp >30°C; double dosing interval above 30°C; give maximum of 3 shocks until temp >30°C; remove wet clothing; use blankets; heat ambulance; give warmed IV fluids (40°C) and warmed humidified O_2; aim for temp = 32 to 34°C
• Tension pneumothorax	needle decompression with 12 G cannula
• Cardiac tamponade	thoracotomy if penetrating chest wound and signs of life within 10 min or rapid transportation to surgical facility
• Toxins	specific antidotes / supportive agents - e.g. naloxone for opioids; flumazenil for benzodiazepines; sodium bicarbonate for tricyclics
• Thrombosis / embolism	fluid loading for amniotic fluid embolus/rapid transfer to hospital

N.B. *Never* terminate resuscitation of the pregnant patient in the pre-hospital setting

Figure 11.4   Advanced life support algorithm for obstetric cardiac arrest. (Adapted from Resuscitation Council (UK). *Adult Advanced Life Support Algorithm*. Available at: http://www.resus.org.uk/pages/gl5algos.htm. Accessed 1 August 2008.)

Top tip

Always pre-alert the receiving hospitals' obstetric unit if you are
on route with a seriously ill or injured patient: ideally, speak
directly to the senior obstetrician on call.

Top tip

Remaining on scene after more than 4 minutes of active CPR
with no response will dramatically reduce the probability of
survival for a mother and fetus after 24 weeks of pregnancy.

PERIMORTEM CAESAREAN SECTION

Definition

Perimortem CS is a modified type of CS used after 24 weeks' gestation in cases of maternal cardiopulmonary arrest, when there
has been no response to 4 minutes of active CPR. The prime aim
of perimortem CS is to facilitate maternal resuscitation and maximise the chance of maternal survival. Although fetal survival is
possible, this is not the prime aim of the procedure. Perimortem
CS would still be considered for maternal reasons, even if the baby
was known to have died. The nearer to term (37 weeks or more)
that the incident has occurred, the better the chance of fetal survival. However, it is likely that at any gestation beyond 24 weeks
(5–6 months), the option of perimortem Caesarean would be
considered.

All causes of maternal collapse may lead to cardiopulmonary
arrest. One of the most common is major obstetric haemorrhage.
Whatever the cause, active CPR with left lateral tilt of 15–30° must
be commenced and maintained until the patient is resuscitated or
until arrival in the hospital setting. There is no place for pausing or
ceasing active CPR as this will compromise the chances of maternal
and fetal survival.

There is little published evidence to base practice on. However, physiology would suggest that perimortem CS should be
commenced after 4 minutes of active CPR if there is no maternal response. Ideally, it should be accomplished within 5 minutes.
Both maternal and fetal survival are maximised if these times can
be accomplished. In one review, 70% of fetuses delivered within
5 minutes survived neurologically intact. Obviously with an arrest
in the pre-hospital setting, achieving these times is very unlikely.

However, there are reported cases of intact fetal survival when perimortem CS has been started more than 20 minutes after the arrest. Although maternal outcome is extremely poor with delayed perimortem CS, the fetal data should encourage maintenance of CPR throughout transfer. The transfer should also be undertaken as rapidly as possible.

Risk factors
- any cause of maternal collapse resulting in cardiopulmonary arrest
- obesity is a particular risk factor implicated in many causes of maternal collapse

Diagnosis
Use standard assessment techniques to diagnose maternal cardiac arrest and institute active CPR. Perimortem CS should be considered for all causes of cardiac arrest in late pregnancy, when active CPR has not led to signs of recovery within 4 minutes. An awareness of this timescale will encourage rapid transfer from the pre-hospital setting.

Top tip

Rapid transfer to hospital with continuous CPR is recommended in cases of maternal cardiac arrest after 24 weeks' gestation.

Pre-hospital management
1 institute active CPR with 15–30° of left lateral tilt
2 proceed with rapid transfer (lights and sirens) to an emergency department in a hospital with senior obstetric staff on site
3 inform hospital – remember to ask for a senior obstetrician to be present on arrival
4 continue active CPR without pausing during transfer
5 if IV access has not been secured – consider gaining access during transfer

---

Top tip

When active CPR has been started in the pre-hospital setting, ask for a senior obstetrician to be present at the predicted time of arrival at hospital.

> **Box 11.2: Steps in perimortem CS (this should only be carried out by an appropriately qualified doctor IN HOSPITAL)**
>
> **1** Decision to proceed to CS – continue active CPR.
> **2** Prepare for possible neonatal resuscitation.
> **3** Wear sterile gloves and apply basic skin preparation.
> **4** Anaesthetist is not required (patient has arrested).
> **5** Rapid entry – appropriate incision in abdominal wall and uterus.
> **6** Deliver baby – hand over for assessment and possible resuscitation.
> **7** Leave placenta in place – bleeding is minimal because of cardiac arrest.
> **8** Open cardiac massage via the diaphragm may be considered with the abdomen open.
> **9** If resuscitation is successful, anaesthetist will administer general anaesthesia.
> **10** Deliver placenta and close uterus and abdominal wall.

The steps in perimortem CS are included as additional information in Box 11.2. The surgical technique for undertaking perimortem CS requires little in the way of formal instrumentation. The most important issue is making the decision to proceed.

SHOCK IN PREGNANCY

Definition
Shock can be defined as a failure of perfusion of the tissues with oxygenated blood. This may be due to loss of circulating fluid volume due to haemorrhage (hypovolaemic shock), movement of circulating fluid volume into the interstitial spaces due to increased capillary permeability (septic shock), pump failure or obstruction in the circulatory system (cardiogenic shock), severe allergic reaction (anaphylactic shock), disruption of the nervous system (neurogenic shock), or severe stress (psychogenic shock).

Risk factors
- inter-current heart disease (cardiogenic shock)
- thromboembolism and amniotic fluid embolism (cardiogenic shock)
- non-obstetric infections and genital tract sepsis (septic shock)

- trauma (hypovolaemic shock)
- obstetric haemorrhage (hypovolaemic shock)
- inverted uterus (neurogenic or hypovolaemic shock)
- ruptured ectopic pregnancy (hypovolaemic shock)
- incomplete miscarriage (neurogenic or hypovolaemic shock)
- opiate-induced histamine release or other drug allergy (anaphylaxis)

Diagnosis

> **Top tip**
>
> The normal physiological changes of pregnancy (increased plasma and red cell volume) allow the patient to compensate for some time. This can make diagnosis difficult as changes in vital signs may be minimal. Always have a high index of suspicion for concealed internal haemorrhage.

In postpartum haemorrhage (PPH) and trauma to the genital tract external haemorrhage will be obvious and the volume of blood seen may give an indication of the amount of blood lost. However, even in PPH some of the bleeding may be concealed.

In ruptured ectopic pregnancy and placental abruption almost all of the blood lost may be internal and concealed. As patients in pregnancy will initially compensate for hypovolaemia, the pre-hospital practitioner must obtain a good history which may, if abnormal, form the basis of a suspicion that concealed haemorrhage may be present.

See Table 11.1 for a summary of the differential diagnosis of shock in the obstetric patient.

> **Top tip**
>
> The main mechanism of maintaining maternal circulation in the event of blood loss is the restriction of blood flow to the uterus. This can occur rapidly following the onset of significant bleeding, and will result in a reduction in placental perfusion with associated fetal hypoxia. Consequently, even in the absence of signs of shock, control of haemorrhage and restoration of circulating volume have the highest priority.

Pre-hospital management

General principles

1 Remember to position the mother in the 15–30° left lateral position to avoid further compromise of the fetal circulation due to vena caval compression by the uterus.

Table 11.1   Differential diagnosis of shock in the obstetric patient.

Aetiology	Pulse rate	BP	Gestation	Blood loss	Other key features
Ruptured ectopic	↑	↓	First trimester (but may not know they are pregnant)	+++ (but probably concealed)	Peritonism; consider possibility in **any** woman of childbearing years with unexplained shock and abdominal pain
Cervical shock	↓	↓	Usually first trimester	+	History suggestive of miscarriage
APH	↑	↓	Second and third trimester	+++ (but may be concealed)	Known placenta praevia; trauma to abdomen, possibly woody uterus
Uterine rupture	↑or↓	↓	Labour	+++ (but may be concealed)	History of uterine surgery (C-section, fibroids); abdominal trauma
AFE	↑	↓	Advanced or rapid labour	None	Suspect in any patient in advanced labour with sudden collapse including hypoxia and cardiovascular compromise in the absence of any other likely diagnosis
Uterine inversion	↓	↓	Third stage of labour	+	Visible uterus at introitus; may have resulted from cord traction ('managed third stage')
PPH	↑	↓	Postpartum	+ to +++	Primary PPH associated with perineal and vaginal trauma; secondary PPH may be associated with sepsis; either may be associated with retained placenta/parts
Anaphylaxis	↑	↓	Any	None	Allergen related (history of atopy); may be drug related – think morphine/opiates

2 Open, maintain and protect the airway in accordance with the patient's clinical need.

3 If oxygen saturation on air falls below 94% give oxygen. If SpO_2 is less than 85% use non-rebreathing mask; otherwise use a simple face mask. Aim for a target saturation of 94–98%.

4 Start transportation without delay to a hospital with obstetric theatres, blood transfusion, ICU and anaesthetic services immediately available.

5 Inform the senior on-call obstetrician of your impending arrival.

6 Insert two large-bore (14 G) cannulae on route (do NOT delay on scene to do this). If it is not possible to gain IV access, consider using an intraosseous cannula.

7 In hypovolaemia, septic shock, neurogenic shock and anaphylaxis only: administer crystalloids in 250 ml aliquots to maintain a systolic BP of 100 mm Hg. Withhold fluids if the SBP is 100 mm Hg or above to reduce the risk of re-bleeding due to clot disruption unless there is other evidence of significant haemorrhage, such as:
- more than 500 ml of external haemorrhage or
- altered mental status
- dysrhythmias

8 Administer analgesia if the patient is in pain – use morphine cautiously if the patient is hypotensive.

9 Give nothing by mouth as the patient is likely to require anaesthesia and surgery (see Fig. 11.5 for the complete shock algorithm).

Top tip

In the pre-hospital setting excessive intravenous fluids should be avoided in cases of cardiogenic shock as administration can cause fluid overload and worsen pulmonary oedema.

Specific management

Cardiogenic shock: provide supportive treatment – treat dysrhythmias according to usual Resuscitation Council (UK) guidelines.

Anaphylactic shock: treat in accordance with normal pre-hospital guidelines:
- oxygen via non-rebreathing mask
- adrenaline 0.5 mg IM repeated once only
- salbutamol 5 mg nebulisers to treat wheeze
- hydrocortisone 200 mg slow IV injection
- chlorpheniramine 10 mg slow IV injection

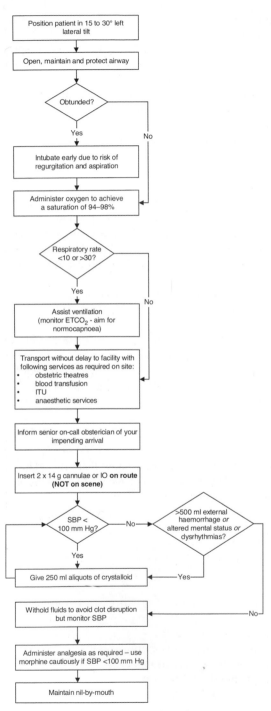

Figure 11.5 Universal shock algorithm.

- IV crystalloids to maintain blood pressure
- adrenaline 1:100,000 infusion IV as a last resort (experienced practitioners only)

Top tip

Opioids, including morphine, cause histamine release: in a small proportion of patients this can lead to anaphylactic reactions.

Top tip

Spending time **on-scene** to cannulate and give fluids to a haemorrhaging obstetric patient wastes time and reduces the probability of survival for the mother and fetus.

Top tip

The most effective treatment of obstetric haemorrhage is usually surgery in an appropriately equipped and staffed maternity theatre suite.

SUMMARY OF KEY POINTS

In cardiac arrest:
- Resuscitation following maternal cardiac arrest should always be commenced and never terminated in the pre-hospital setting, even if the probability of survival for the mother is minimal, to maximise the chances of survival for both the mother and the fetus.
- Cardiac arrest victims beyond 24 weeks of pregnancy must NOT be managed in the supine position. Instead they should be secured to a spine board tilted 15–30° to the patient's left.
- Tracheal intubation, using Sellick's manoeuvre, must be performed as quickly as possible to minimise the risk of aspiration.
- Ventilation of the obtunded pregnant patient must always be via a cuffed airway device.
- Ventilation to compression ratios, defibrillation electrode placement and energy settings, and drug doses are the same for obstetric patients as non-pregnant patient.
- The most common presenting cardiac arrest rhythm in pregnancy is PEA.

- The decision to move the patient must be taken early in the resuscitation attempt to permit emergency perimortem CS and maximise the probability of maternal and fetal survival.
- Spending time on-scene to cannulate and give fluids to a haemorrhaging obstetric patient wastes time and reduces the probability of survival of the mother and fetus.
- CPR should be continued throughout transfer to hospital where the decision to proceed to perimortem Caesarean will be made.
- When informing the hospital about the transfer, remember to recommend that an obstetrician should be in attendance when you arrive at the hospital.

In shock:

- The normal physiological changes of pregnancy (increased plasma and red cell volume) allow the patient to compensate for some time. This can make diagnosis difficult as changes in vital signs may be minimal. Always have a high index of suspicion for concealed internal haemorrhage.
- The main mechanism of maintaining maternal circulation in the event of blood loss is the restriction of blood flow to the uterus. This can occur rapidly following the onset of significant bleeding, and will result in a reduction in placental perfusion with associated fetal hypoxia. Consequently, even in the absence of signs of shock, control of haemorrhage and restoration of circulating volume have the highest priority.
- In the haemorrhaging obstetric patient use 250 ml aliquots of crystalloid to maintain a systolic blood pressure of 100 mm Hg.
- In the pre-hospital setting intravenous fluids should be avoided in cases of cardiogenic shock as administration can cause fluid overload and worsen pulmonary oedema.
- Opioids, including morphine, cause histamine release: in a small proportion of patients this can lead to anaphylactic reactions.
- The most effective treatment of obstetric haemorrhage is usually surgery in an appropriately equipped and staffed maternity theatre suite.

Abbreviations

OBSTETRIC ABBREVIATIONS

The following obstetric abbreviations may be seen within the woman's hand-held notes and are used by both obstetricians and midwives. This list is not exhaustive. Full definitions can be found in the Glossary.

AFE	amniotic fluid embolism
AFLP	acute fatty liver of pregnancy
AFP	alfa feta protein
A/N	antenatal
APH	antepartum haemorrhage
BBA	born before arrival
Br	breech
CS	Caesarean section
Cx	cervix
Ceph	cephalic
EDD	estimated date of delivery
EFD	early fetal demise
EL	elective (referring to CS)
EM	emergency (referring to CS)
FHHR	fetal heart heard and regular
FMF	fetal movements felt
FMNF	fetal movements not felt
HELLP	haemolysis-elevated liver enzymes and low platelets
G	gravidity
IUD	intrauterine death
IOL	induction of labour
LMP	last menstrual period
LSCS	lower section Caesarean section
MW	midwife
NND	neonatal death
OBS	obstetrics
P	parity
PHR	patient held records

PN	postnatal
PPH	postpartum haemorrhage
Prem	premature/preterm
RPOC	retained products of conception
SROM	spontaneous rupture of membranes
Vx	vertex

Glossary

OBSTETRIC TERMINOLOGY

The following obstetric terminology and abbreviations may be seen within the woman's hand-held notes, and are used by both obstetricians and midwives. Some hand-held notes list some of this terminology and its meaning in the front of the notes for the use of women and their partners. The following list is not exhaustive, but endeavours to cover the more commonly used terminology and abbreviations.

36 + 5: 36 weeks and 5 days pregnant.

5:10: 5 contractions in 10 minutes (= hyperstimulation).

A

Accoucher: French for a male obstetrician, a physician skilled in the art and science of managing pregnancy, labour and the puerperium (the time after delivery).

Active third stage: Delivery of the placenta using drugs and controlled cord traction to deliver the placenta.

Acute fatty liver of pregnancy (AFLP): Liver failure in late pregnancy, usually from unknown cause.

Amniotic fluid embolism (AFE): Entry of liquor into the maternal circulation. A rare cause of maternal collapse.

Ampullary pregnancy: Ectopic pregnancy in the outer, wider part of the fallopian tube.

Antenatal (A/N) or Antepartum: Events before birth.

Antepartum haemorrhage (APH): Bleeding from the birth canal before birth and after 24 weeks' gestation.

Apgar score: A system used to assess the condition of the baby during the first few minutes of birth.

Alfa feta protein (AFP): One of the blood tests used to screen for Down's syndrome in the fetus.

B

Bicornuate uterus: Having two horns or horn-shaped branches. The uterus (normally unicornuate) can sometimes be bicornuate

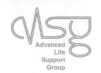

(with two branches, e.g. one at about 10:30 and the other at about 1:30).

Born before arrival (BBA): Unplanned delivery of the baby outside the hospital environment.

Breech presentation: Buttocks of the infant in the lower pole of the uterus.

C

Caesarean section: Often referred to as **CS** (Caesarean section) or **LSCS** (lower segment caesarean section; em = emergency, el = elective).

Cervix (Cx): Lower portion of the neck of the uterus.

Cephalic (Ceph): The fetal head. May also be known as the **Vertex (Vx)**.

Cord prolapse: When the membranes rupture and a cord is presenting in front of the fetus.

D

Dystocia: Means "difficult." May be associated with shoulder dystocia, or labour dystocia (protracted labour).

E

Early pregnancy: Pregnancies up to 24 weeks, especially before 20 weeks.

Early pregnancy assessment unit: Direct access for the management of women with early pregnancy problems.

Ectopic pregnancy: A pregnancy developing outside the uterus, usually in the fallopian tubes.

ECV: External cephalic version – method of turning a baby from the breech position to head down position.

Estimated date of delivery (EDD): This is initially based on the LMP then from a 12-week dating scan.

Engagement: Entry of the presenting part of the fetus (usually head) into the pelvis.

Episiotomy: A surgical incision made into the perineum to enlarge the vaginal orifice.

F

Fetus: The unborn baby.

Fetal heart heard and regular (FHHR): Documented following auscultation of the fetal heart.

Fetal movements felt (FMF): Documented following enquiring about, or observing fetal movements.

Fetal movements not felt (FMNF): Documented in the notes when a mother has not yet felt movements in early pregnancy or when movements cannot be felt in late pregnancy. This may be associated with fetal death.

G

Gestation or gestational age: The completed weeks of pregnancy (not months). The mother's dates are usually calculated from the 12-week dating scan rather than the **last menstrual period (LMP)**. This will give a more accurate **expected date of delivery (EDD)**.

Gravid: Pregnant.

Gravidity (G) (also see parity): The number of times a woman has been pregnant, including the current pregnancy. This is regardless of the outcome of the pregnancies (for example it includes miscarriages).

H

Haemolysis-elevated liver enzymes and low platelets (HELLP): A syndrome featuring a combination of 'H' for haemolysis (the breakdown of red blood cells), 'EL' for elevated liver enzymes and 'LP' for low platelet count (an essential blood clotting element).

Hyperstimulation: More than five contractions in 10 minutes.

I

Intrapartum: Events during labour.

Intrauterine: Within the uterus. For example, intrauterine transfer – transfer of a woman still pregnant.

Intrauterine death (IUD): Death of the fetus within the uterus.

Induction of labour (IOL): Labour that is artificially induced by various means.

Isthmus: Narrow middle portion of the fallopian tube.

Introitus: Entrance to the vagina

L

Labour: Childbirth is described in three stages.

Lie: The relationship between the long axis of the fetus to the uterus. This may be longitudinal, transverse or oblique.

Liquor: The fluid which fills then amniotic sac surrounding the baby.

Lithotomy: Position in which the patient is on their back with the hips and knees flexed and the thighs apart. The position is often used for vaginal examinations and childbirth.

Livebirth: A baby born alive, irrespective of gestational age.

Lochia: The discharge from the uterus following childbirth, consisting of blood.

M

Meconium: Bright or dark green material which may be expelled from the fetal bowel whilst still in utero. It may be evident when

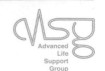

woman's waters have broken. It will be expelled from the baby following delivery.

Midwife (MW): A practitioner responsible for providing midwifery care to women during the antenatal, intrapartum and postnatal periods.

Miscarriage: the expulsion of the products of a pregnancy (in whole or part) before the end of the 24th week of pregnancy. It is associated with vaginal bleeding and pain. The term **early fetal demise (EFD)** is now also used.

Multigravida (or Multip): A pregnant woman who is not in her first pregnancy. A grand multip is a woman who has had a minimum of five births.

Multiple pregnancy: Pregnancy with more than one fetus.

N

Neonatal: The newborn baby.

Neonatal death (NND): Death of a live born baby within 28 days.

O

Obstetrics (Obs): A branch of medicine dealing with pregnancy, labour and the puerperium.

Occiput: The back of the fetal head.

P

Parity (P) (see also gravidity): Refers to the number of live births plus stillbirths a woman has had. For example, you may see **G3 P2** written. This means that this woman is in her third pregnancy, and has had two births. **G5 P2** means that the woman is in her fifth pregnancy but has only had two live births. The other two pregnancies may have been miscarriages.

Pathway of care: This can be either high, or low risk.

Patient held records (PHR): Hand-held maternity notes that the woman carries with her throughout her pregnancy.

Perinatal: Around the time of birth.

Physiological second stage: Natural, without the use of drugs and controlled cord traction.

Placental location: Describes the relationship of the placenta in the uterus. It can be anterior, posterior, fundal, lateral or low. There are various ways of describing a low lying placenta or praevia – distance from the internal cervical os (usually given in mm), partially covering os or completely covering the os, or major or minor placenta praevia.

Position: Referring to position of the baby in the uterus, using the fetal occiput as the denominator, for example occipito-anterior and occipito-posterior.

Postnatal (PN): After childbirth.

Postpartum: After labour.

Postpartum haemorrhage (PPH): 'Primary' PPH means blood loss of more than 500 ml from the birth canal within 24 hours of delivery. 'Secondary' PPH means excessive bleeding more than 24 hours after delivery.

Presentation: The part of the baby which will be delivered first. For example, cephalic (head) or breech (buttocks).

Precipitate labour: A labour that is very fast. **A precipitate delivery** is therefore a rapid delivery.

Premature or preterm (Prem): Referring to labour or delivery before 37 completed weeks of gestation.

Primigravida (Primip): A woman in her first pregnancy.

Puerperium: The 6-week period after the birth of the baby during which the mother's reproductive organs return to their pre-pregnant state.

R

Retained products of conception (RPOC): Products of conception refers to the combination of fetal and placental tissue.

S

Spontaneous rupture of the membranes (SROM): When the 'waters break'.

Stillbirth (SB): A baby born after 24 weeks showing NO SIGNS OF LIFE at delivery. The fetus may have died days or even weeks before within the uterus. HOWEVER, a baby of any gestation which shows signs of life has to be registered as a LIVE BIRTH. If you are involved with a pre-hospital birth in these circumstances, you must inform the relevant midwife and obstetrician.

T

Term: When pregnancy is completed within 37–42 weeks.

Trimester: A period of 3 months.

Tubal abortion: A term applied to an ectopic pregnancy when the conceptus is extruded from the fimbrial end of the fallopian tube.

V

Viability: The ability of the fetus to survive independently. Legally this is from 24 weeks' gestation.

References

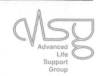

Support
Group

Life

Advanced

ALSO. Advanced Life Support in Obstetrics Provider Manual, 4th edn. Kansas: American Academy of Family Physicians; 2004.

Beveridge CJE, Wilkinson AR. Sodium bicarbonate infusion during resuscitation of infants at birth. Cochrane Review in The Cochrane Library, Issue 1, 2006. Available at: http://www.thecochrane library .com.

Bolam v. Friern Hospital Management Committee. 1, WLR 582; 1957.

Boyle M. Emergencies Around Childbirth: A Handbook for Midwives, 2nd edn. Buckingham: Open University press; 2002.

Byrne S, Fisher S, Fortune P-M, Lawn C, Wieteska S. Paediatric and Neonatal Safe Transfer and Retrieval: The Practical Approach. Oxford: Advanced Life Support Group, Blackwell-Wiley; 2008.

Cheng M, Hannah M. Breech delivery at term: a critical review of the literature. Obstet Gynecol 1993;82:605–18.

Confidential Enquiry into Maternal and Child Health. Why Mothers Die 2000–2002. Report on confidential enquiries into maternal deaths in the United Kingdom. London: CEMACH; 2004.

Confidential Enquiry into Maternal and Child Health. Diabetes in Pregnancy: Are We Providing the Best Care? Findings of a National Enquiry: England, Wales and Northern Ireland. London: CEMACH; 2007a.

Confidential Enquiry into Maternal and Child Health. Perinatal Mortality. 2005: England, Wales and Northern Ireland. London: CEMACH; 2007b.

Confidential Enquiry into Maternal and Child Health. Why Mothers Die 2003–2005. Report on confidential enquiries into maternal deaths in the United Kingdom. London: CEMACH; 2007c.

Cox C, Grady K. Managing Obstetric Emergencies. Oxford: Bios publishing Ltd.; 2002.

Crown Prosecution Service. Policy for Prosecuting Cases of Rape. London: CPS Communications Branch; March 2009.

Data Protection Act. London: Information Commissioner's Office; 1998.

Dawson A, Subak-Sharpe R, Woollard M. Obstetrics and gynaecology. In: IHCD (eds). Ambulance Service Paramedic Training. Bristol: IHCD; 1999.

Department of Health. National Service Framework for Diabetes: Standards. London: DH; 2001.

Department of Health. NHS Maternity Stats for England 2004–2005. London: DH; 2006.

Dobbie AE, Cooke MW. A descriptive review and discussion of litigation claims against ambulance services. Emerg Med J 2008;25(7):455–8.

Driscoll P, Macartney I, Mackway-Jones K, Metcalfe E, Oakley P. Safe Transfer and Retrieval of Patients (STAR): The Practical Approach. Oxford: Advanced Life Support Group, Blackwell-Wiley; 2006.

Elbourne D, Chalmers I, Waterhouse I, Holt E. The Newbury maternity care study: a randomized controlled trial to assess a policy of women holding their own obstetric records. Br J Obstet Gynaecol 1987;94: 612–19.

Hanna NJ, Black M, Sander JW, Smithson WH, Appleton R, Brown S, Fish DR. The National Sentinel Clinical Audit of Epilepsy-Related Death: Epilepsy – Death in the Shadows. London: The Stationery Office; 2002.

Hannah ME. Planned Caesarean section versus planned vaginal birth for breech presentation at term: randomised Multicentre trial. The Lancet 2000;356(9239).

Health Professions Council. Standards of Conduct, Performance and Ethics. London: Health Professions Council; 2008.

Johanson J, Cox C, Grady K, Howell C. Managing Obstetric Emergencies and Trauma: The MOET Course Manual. London: RCOG Press; 2003.

Murphy VE, Gibson P, Talbot PI, Clifton VL. Severe asthma exacerbations during pregnancy. Obstet Gynecol 2005;106:1046–54.

National Institute for Health and Clinical Excellence. CG45 Antenatal and Postnatal Mental Health; NICE Guideline. London: NICE; 2007.

Pritchard JA, MacDonald PC. Dystocia Caused by Abnormalities in Presentation, Position or Development of the Fetus. Williams Obstetrics. Norwalk, CT: Appleton-Century-Crofts; 1980, pp 787–96.

Rey E, Boulet LP. Asthma in pregnancy. BMJ 2007;334:582–5.

Royal College of Obstetricians and Gynaecologists Clinical Audit Unit. Effective Procedures in Maternity Care Suitable for Audit. London: RCOG Press; 1997, p. 32. 4.7. Breech presentation at term.

Royal College of Obstetricians and Gynaecologists. Thromboembolic Disease in Pregnancy and the Puerperium: Acute Management. Guideline no 28. London: RCOG Press; 2001.

Sethupathi M. Neonatal outcome after cord prolapse at term (online). Available at: http://www.bwhct.nhs.uk/bwm09001.htm. Accessed 5 July 2007.

Heslehurst N, Ells LJ, Batterham A, Wilkinson J, Summerbell CD. Trends in maternal obesity incidence rates, demographic predictors and health inequalities in 36821 women over 15 years. BJOG 2007;114:187–94.

UKOSS. Annual Report; 2007.

Uygur D, Kis S, Tuncer R, Ozcan FS, Erkaya S. Risk factors and infant outcomes associated with umbilical cord prolapse [Abstract]. Int J Gynaecol Obstet 2002;78(2):127–30.

Woollard M, Simpson H, Hinshaw K, Wieteska S. Training for prehospital obstetric emergencies. Emerg Med J 2008;25(7):392–3.

Woollard M, Todd I. Legal issues. In: Greaves I, Porter K, Hodgetts T, Woollard M (eds). Emergency Care: A Textbook for Paramedics, 2nd edn. Edinburgh: Saunders Elsevier; 2006.

FURTHER READING
Grady K, Howell C, Cox C (eds). The Managing Obstetric Emergencies and Trauma Course Manual, 2nd edn. London: RCOG Press; 2007.

Index

Note: Italicised b, f, and t refer to boxes, figures and tables

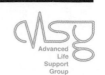
Advanced
Life
Support
Group

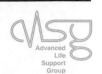

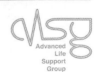

Advanced
Life
Support
Group

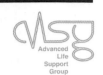

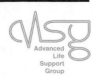

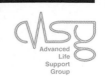